STOPPING PAIN

A Simple, Revolutionary Way to Beat Chronic Pain

BY **JOHNATHAN EDWARDS, MD**
FOREWORD BY **BERNARD GUEZ, MD**

Skyhorse Publishing

Copyright © 2025 by Johnathan Edwards, MD

All rights reserved. No part of this book may be reproduced in any manner without the express written consent of the publisher, except in the case of brief excerpts in critical reviews or articles. All inquiries should be addressed to Skyhorse Publishing, 307 West 36th Street, 11th Floor, New York, NY 10018.

Skyhorse Publishing books may be purchased in bulk at special discounts for sales promotion, corporate gifts, fund-raising, or educational purposes. Special editions can also be created to specifications. For details, contact the Special Sales Department, Skyhorse Publishing, 307 West 36th Street, 11th Floor, New York, NY 10018 or info@skyhorsepublishing.com.

Skyhorse® and Skyhorse Publishing® are registered trademarks of Skyhorse Publishing, Inc.®, a Delaware corporation.

Visit our website at www.skyhorsepublishing.com.

10 9 8 7 6 5 4 3 2 1

Library of Congress Cataloging-in-Publication Data is available on file.

Cover design by David Ter-Avanesyan
Cover illustration: Getty Images

ISBN: 978-1-5107-8342-3
Ebook ISBN: 978-1-5107-8361-4

Printed in the United States of America

Contents

Author's Note v
Prologue vii
Introduction: Stopping Chronic Pain ix
Foreword xiii
How to Use This book xvii

Part One: The Problem

Chapter 1: The Problem with Pain 3
Chapter 2: Medicine in a Changing World 22
Chapter 3: A New Way of Thinking about Medicine—Percutaneous Hydrotomy 42

Part Two: The Science

Chapter 4: The Five Foundations of Percutaneous Hydrotomy 65
Chapter 5: How Percutaneous Hydrotomy Works and Its Physiologic Basis 86
Chapter 6: The Fundamental Techniques of Percutaneous Hydrotomy 104
Chapter 7: How Percutaneous Hydrotomy Treats Common Conditions 114

Part Three: The Future—Percutaneous Hydrotomy and You

Chapter 8: Percutaneous Hydrotomy and the Future 141

Chapter 9: Giving the Floor to the Patients: Testimonials 155

Chapter 10: How to Find a Clinic and Common Questions 180

References 187
Index 218
About the Author 220

Author's Note

The stories in this book are true. Individual names and identifying characteristics of the individuals in the stories have been changed to protect their privacy. Every effort has been made to ensure the information in this book is complete and accurate. However, because of the rapidly evolving nature of regenerative medicine, the authors, publishers, and all other persons and entities associated with this book cannot guarantee the accuracy of all information contained herein. This book's ideas, procedures, and suggestions are not intended as a substitute for consulting with your physician. All matters regarding your health require careful, thoughtful, individual medical supervision. The authors, the publishers, or any other person or entity associated with them or with this book or mentioned herein shall not be liable or responsible for any loss or damage allegedly arising from any information, case studies, therapies, recommendations, suggestions, or anything else in this book or from information readers obtained from websites, articles, books, organizations, healthcare providers, or other medical practitioners mentioned in this book.

At the time of this writing, no formal residencies are available in regenerative injection techniques, mesotherapy, percutaneous hydrotomy, or integrative orthopedic medicine. Hence any physician licensed as a medical or osteopathic physician can legally perform these procedures, as well as many other healthcare providers. The authors strongly recommend that healthcare providers only perform these procedures after sufficient education, training, and experience. No person associated with this book is responsible if a reader seeks help from an insufficiently trained healthcare provider.

Patients desiring any of the treatments described in this book should carefully consider seeking out the recommendations of the organizations and studies cited, which have a long track record of doing research and training in these fields.

Prologue

Chronic pain is as real as it gets. Living with pain is a reality for millions of people and the number continues to rise, not fall. Unfortunately, treatments for chronic pain have not kept up with demand. However, regenerative injection techniques for chronic pain have become mainstream and serve as a crucial bridge between conventional treatments, providing relief to individuals suffering from chronic conditions that previously had limited options for relief. Percutaneous (*per·cu·ta·ne·ous*) hydrotomy is a regenerative injection technique that has been used in Europe for decades. The term is challenging, but it's a revolutionary approach to beating chronic pain and increasing function.

Dr. Johnathan Edwards found percutaneous hydrotomy in a fortuitous chain of events—or, some might say it found him. He was the first American physician to complete his training in percutaneous hydrotomy with Dr. Bernard Guez and bring the technique to the United States. Because percutaneous hydrotomy has traditionally been taught in French, only a handful of English-speaking physicians have been trained. Dr. Edwards, fluent in French, developed a keen interest in the techniques and has been treating patients with percutaneous hydrotomy for several years.

Stopping Pain

He presented the case of a well-known UFC fighter, T.J. Dillashaw, at the 2021 International Society of Percutaneous Hydrotomy (ISPH) meeting in Nice, France. Dr. Edwards now teaches percutaneous hydrotomy techniques in the United States, fulfilling a lifelong ambition for Dr. Guez.

Dr. Edwards has performed percutaneous hydrotomy on thousands of patients. In the following pages, you will find several case examples illustrating the healing aspects of percutaneous hydrotomy. Dr. Edwards has treated many professional athletes using percutaneous hydrotomy, including NFL players, UFC athletes, motocross racers, cyclists, and professional tennis players. These world-class athletes have been able to compete again after sidelining injuries and have returned to regular active lives. Most importantly, you will read numerous patient testimonials from people afflicted with chronic disease who regained their lives after percutaneous hydrotomy treatments.

This book was written with the goal of increasing interest in percutaneous hydrotomy in the United States and other English-speaking countries. In conjunction with Dr. Guez and the ISHP, Dr. Edwards has trained many practitioners in the art and science of percutaneous hydrotomy.

Introduction: Stopping Chronic Pain

This book introduces a groundbreaking paradigm shift in the treatment of musculoskeletal injuries and chronic pain. It delves into pioneering medical treatments that have the potential to significantly alter outcomes for individuals dealing with chronic pain. While hundreds of thousands of patients have already benefited from these treatments, they remain relatively unknown to many patients and underutilized by healthcare providers. These innovative techniques harness the body's own healing capabilities to establish a connection between traditional standard-of-care treatments for musculoskeletal injuries. Importantly, the methods described in this book are cost-effective and minimally invasive, especially in comparison to surgical procedures. Paradoxically, they aren't covered by insurance, even though their utilization could potentially save billions within the healthcare system.

Numerous patients have experienced positive results from the procedures detailed in this book, which aims to provide essential information about integrative general medicine and orthopedics to the millions of individuals who suffer from chronic pain and other debilitating conditions. This book seeks to educate patients about various often superior alternatives to currently employed treatments and medications. The new paradigm presented in this book has the potential to revolutionize the treatment of chronic pain.

Chronic pain is a widespread issue, with the number of individuals in the United States diagnosed with osteoarthritis rising dramatically. Lower back pain has been labeled as the "disease of the century." These costs, affecting both individuals and society, are expected to rise due to the increasing prevalence of obesity, the diabetes epidemic, and a decrease in recreational activity.

In the United States, over half a million prosthetic knees are implanted each year. However, many patients aren't suitable candidates for these highly invasive procedures, and those who are often endure years of pain waiting for insurance approval. While surgery successfully addresses many medical conditions like diseased cartilage, tendons, and ligaments, it can exacerbate osteoarthritis.

Standard conservative treatments for musculoskeletal injuries and chronic pain typically involve medications, physical therapy, activity modifications, bracing, steroid injections, and, if all else fails, surgery. Until regenerative injection therapies gained mainstream acceptance, patients had few alternatives. Regenerative injection treatments form the basis of this new paradigm. Collectively, these therapies can assist with acute and chronic injuries to tendons, bones, ligaments, and cartilage, and they can also alleviate or eliminate arthritic joint pain.

At the time of this writing, regenerative injection therapies include prolotherapy, platelet-rich plasma injections (PRP), stem cell injections, perineural injections, and saline injections. This book primarily focuses on percutaneous hydrotomy, another type of regenerative technique.

Introduction: Stopping Chronic Pain

Prolotherapy, dating back to the 1930s, involves a series of injections using saline, local anesthetics, dextrose, or other tissue-stimulating (proliferant) solutions. These injections induce inflammation and the release of growth factors, activating the body's immune system to initiate the healing process. Most patients experience a positive difference after a few treatments.

Platelet-rich plasma treatment, or PRP, is widely used by top athletes and patients worldwide and has received extensive coverage in major newspapers worldwide. PRP involves taking the patient's blood and separating and concentrating platelets and then injecting them into the target area using precise medical injection techniques. Platelets contain numerous growth factors that signal stem cells to promote cartilage and soft tissue repair, reduce inflammation, stimulate bone grafting, enhance wound healing, and minimize blood loss. While this treatment may require several days of downtime and up to six weeks away from intense training, many athletes have reported faster recovery.

Adult stem cell injections typically involve using stem cells harvested from the patient's own bone marrow, cells, or fat cells, or the human placenta, which are all rich in stem cells. These cells are prepared and then injected into injured or degenerated areas. Although relatively new, this method holds promise, particularly for the treatment of advanced arthritis, severely degenerated tendons and ligaments, and chronic pain.

Perineural superficial injection treatment, or PSI, generally involves superficial injections of low-dose dextrose and lidocaine. PSI has proven effective in treating pain caused by irritated or entrapped nerves and conditions like Achilles tendinitis.

The fifth type of regenerative injections involves saline. It may come as a surprise, but simply injecting saline (water) into a painful area can offer relief. Historical records have indicated for centuries that water has healing properties. A multitude of studies support the therapeutic use of saline. The book will provide detailed insights into how water can heal diseased cells.

Regenerative injection techniques serve as a crucial bridge between all conventional treatments, and they provide relief to individuals suffering from chronic conditions that previously had limited options for relief. The book raises questions about the limited adoption of these regenerative injection techniques and why the healthcare system doesn't cover them. *Stopping Pain* aims to educate individuals on regenerative healing and navigating treatment options effectively. The foundation and philosophy of this book is that treating the root causes of pain is fundamental in stopping chronic pain and regaining function.

Foreword by Dr. Bernard Guez

I am a general practitioner, mesotherapist, geriatrician, and aesthetic doctor. After earning my medical degree in France, I pursued a fellowship in mesotherapy at the Sainte Marguerite hospital in Marseille in 1981 under the direction of Dr. Bernard Sauvigné. I also served as an expert in France for the Haute Autorité de Santé, equivalent to being an expert for the medical boards that govern medical specialties. I've been practicing medicine for nearly forty years, have performed nearly 350,000 general medicine interventions, and have spent three decades perfecting the procedures outlined in this book.

As a young physician in the 1980s, I was frequently confronted with patients suffering from chronic diseases such as osteoarthritis, migraines, neuralgias, allergies, ear, nose, and throat infections (particularly in children), and autoimmune diseases. While symptomatic treatments provided relief from the painful episodes of these diseases, they rarely prevented recurrence; they never addressed the root causes.

Stopping Pain

My interest was piqued by mesotherapy, which appeared to offer the beginnings of a solution to chronic diseases. Mesotherapy involves injecting water, vitamins, and drugs in precise amounts and locations. Over the subsequent fifteen years, I evolved my mesotherapy practice by increasing the use of physiological saline and expanding the areas for injection. By incorporating more water into the treatment to promote healing, I observed improvements in pain management and mobility among my patients. This gave rise to mesotherapy and hydration, a concept that gradually integrated varying amounts of physiologic saline with active ingredients. Depending on the specific chronic disease, I found that using subcutaneous infusions of 10, 20, 50, and even 500 milliliters was effective, safe, and well tolerated. I also noticed that increasing the volume of active ingredients with broader dilutions across larger surface areas improved patient tolerance and the diffusion of the products, yielding even more promising results.

After fifteen years of observation and refinement, I introduced the term "percutaneous hydrotomy" within medical circles. I opted for the term percutaneous hydrotomy because this technique was close to the concept of Dr. Jeffery Klein's tumescent anesthesia technique used since the 1980s for aesthetic medicine. I also discussed this process with Dr. Michel Pistor, the founder of mesotherapy, who strongly encouraged the development of this technique, initially suggesting it be referred to as "surface mesotherapy." In Pistor's book "Practical Mesotherapy", he described my work as marking the dawn of the third millennium. Eventually, I settled on the term "percutaneous hydrotomy."

Results from percutaneous hydrotomy have been nothing short of incredible. Patients have reported a reduction in their pain, an increase in function, an absence of side effects, and the cessation

Foreword by Dr. Bernard Guez

of medications. Above all, they have regained their taste for life. The medical clinic is the best observation post for understanding patients. It gives the medical doctor an inexhaustible source of clues to approaching their care.

In 2006, I established the International Society of Percutaneous Hydrotomy to facilitate the exchange of ideas and teachings among colleagues from various medical disciplines. Each year, during our international congress, numerous healthcare providers share testimonies of the remarkable results they've witnessed in patients who had previously reached therapeutic dead ends.

During the 2020 ISPH meeting, I had the pleasure of meeting Dr. Johnathan Edwards, an American anesthetist who spoke French and showed a keen interest in the technique, even participating in training in France. His lively and intelligent presentations, as well as his unexpected fluency in the French language, impressed us all. It was evident that Dr. Edwards comprehended the therapeutic potential of percutaneous hydrotomy and its applicability in the United States and the English-speaking world.

After multiple discussions and meetings, I am confident that Dr. Edwards is the ideal individual to introduce percutaneous hydrotomy. With his book *Stopping Pain*, he has become a pioneer in the broader application of the concept of percutaneous hydrotomy, offering hope to patients suffering from chronic diseases.

—Bernard Guez, MD

How to Use This Book

This book is designed to be user-friendly and can be approached at different levels. It caters to both patients and healthcare practitioners interested in understanding regenerative injection techniques like percutaneous hydrotomy. Here's how you can make the most of this book.

1. Prospective patients: If you are a patient seeking information about chronic pain, start by reading the patient testimonials. These real-life accounts will provide you with practical insights into how percutaneous hydrotomy can potentially help you in your journey to overcome chronic disease and improve your quality of life.
2. Medical community: You can use this book as part of a study group or discussion. Reading the medical articles in this book will help medical practitioners understand the basis of percutaneous hydrotomy, what it is, and what it is not. Engaging with others can help you gain a broader understanding of the content and share perspectives.
3. Table of contents and index: Refer to the table of contents and index to find information on specific topics that interest

you. This will allow you to navigate the book more efficiently and locate the information you need.
4. Overview: Reading the entire text, including the experiences of Drs. Guez and Edwards, patient testimonials, and the chapters on chronic disease and the origins of percutaneous hydrotomy, will give you a comprehensive overview of what percutaneous hydrotomy entails and its potential benefits.

The book is structured as follows:

- The initial chapters provide insight into the experiences of Dr. Guez and Dr. Edwards and discuss chronic disease's prevalence in today's society.
- The next chapters delve into the origins of percutaneous hydrotomy, exploring the fundamental principles, competencies, and physiological mechanisms underlying this approach.
- Subsequent chapters cover the essential techniques used in percutaneous hydrotomy, the pathophysiology of diseases treatable with this method, and practical applications.
- The book concludes by discussing potential future applications of percutaneous hydrotomy.

A significant highlight of the book is the patient testimonials, which offer powerful accounts of how percutaneous hydrotomy has positively impacted individuals dealing with chronic diseases, helping them regain a zest for life.

Part One
The Problem

CHAPTER 1

The Problem with Pain

Pain is a universal human experience, a visceral and undeniable reality that strikes at the core of our existence. It's an affliction that knows no bias, affecting people from all walks of life; it doesn't matter who you are, the CEO of a large company or someone living in a remote village. While some individuals might possess a remarkable resilience to pain, there's a simple truth: pain is as real as it gets. Regardless of how skeptical or stoic one might be, pain is the common ground where belief is unanimous.

Our contemporary approach to managing chronic pain has fallen short of the mark, and the issue at hand is that many must endure persistent pain, specifically chronic pain. Pain stands as one of the most enigmatic challenges of the human body, a complex riddle with no shortage of purported solutions. Many people who grapple with chronic pain become desperate, resorting to daily medications for survival, only to eventually suffer the secondary effects. Pharmaceutical companies have excelled in creating medications that offer momentary respite from pain, but these drugs do little to address the underlying causes of pain. Worse, they've formulated powerfully addictive painkillers that have caused the loss of millions of lives to overdoses (Abramson, 2022). Despite significant advancements in medical science, the scourge of chronic pain remains, leaving a trail of devastation.

In our world today, pain casts a heavier burden than ever before. Almost half of the global population grapples with chronic illnesses (Zelaya, 2019), encompassing conditions like arthritis, frozen shoulder, back pain, neck pain, degenerative disc disease, sciatica, knee pain, hip pain, migraines, and temporomandibular joint syndrome (TMJ), to name just a few. The magnitude of this statistic is chilling, primarily because the most distressing aspect of chronic pain is the overwhelming isolation it imposes. When a chronic illness diagnosis is received, it fundamentally alters one's life, causing the world to contract. Isolation becomes an insufferable companion, a factor that can lead to despair and even suicide (Edwards, 2023).

There are hundreds of thousands who understand your emotional journey; you are not alone. Those living with chronic diseases or pain encounter distinctive challenges, including the perplexity and isolation that accompany being "differently abled." Chronic disease doesn't happen by chance.

What's Fueling the Chronic Pain Epidemic?

Few ask why. And when doctors pop their heads up for just a second and start asking questions, one quickly realizes what they don't want you to do in healthcare. What's causing the rise of these diseases? Every time we take care of a patient with diabetes or autoimmune disease, there's a voice inside of us whispering, and then a little louder, and finally, with a deafening call, that something is wrong with the American health system. The rise in these diseases

The Problem with Pain

is not just a coincidence, but a result of systemic issues within the American health system.

Presently, suffering with chronic pain is accepted as a normal human condition. We're living in a hyper-fast world, and we throw ourselves into a healthcare system that offers numerous treatment options, but all too often, relief is marginal and sporadic. Surgery, especially for back pain, frequently worsens the problem in the long run. Our contemporary lifestyle encourages poor posture, with regular physical activity becoming a relic of the past, as desks, video games, smartphones, and computers dominate our lives. Humans are meant to move, yet we're moving less, not more. Our access to food is unparalleled in history, but we're consuming addictive foods designed for overconsumption that leave us unsatisfied. This, in turn, leads to obesity, which afflicts over half the population of the United States and is deeply intertwined with the chronic pain epidemic.

Until recent times, most people with chronic pain had to live with the condition or face surgery. The common conservative treatments are activity modification, bracing, medications, psychiatric medications, physical therapy, steroid injections, and weight loss (West, 2020). Once these modalities prove ineffective, pain medications and surgery are the mainstay of treatment. This explains the nearly a million shoulder, hip, and knee replacements that are performed annually in the United States (Williams, 2015). These surgeries also leave patients with the specter of needing another joint replacement within ten to twenty years.

One answer to chronic pain is regenerative medicine. This is a rapidly growing field that aims to treat acute and chronic pain conditions by harnessing the body's natural healing properties to improve function and pain after injury. We've forgotten that our bodies possess an internal resilience to heal. Instead, every problem requires a pill, surgery, or an expert. Miracles happen every day when our bodies heal and perform the many functions essential for life. In modern times, we've ignored this wisdom.

Every healthcare provider has stories of healing that truly amazed them and defied logic. Regenerative injection techniques have existed nearly for a century and are applied locally at the site of injury and work through various mechanisms. They include prolotherapy, platelet-rich plasma (PRP), stem cells, perineural superficial injections (PSI), and saline injections (Yelland, 2004; Linnanmäki, 2020; Simental-Mendía, 2020; Abate, 2018; West, 2020; Shipley, 2013). Chronic diseases like osteoarthritis are particularly amenable to regenerative approaches since patients often fail conservative treatments, ultimately requiring joint replacement to achieve pain relief and improve function and quality of life.

However, some things have changed. For instance, it was once standard of care to prescribe nonsteroidal anti-inflammatory drugs (NSAIDs) like ibuprofen for any type of pain or broken bones. After extensive research, we've circled back with a better understanding that inflammation is a natural part of the healing process and NSAIDs may not be the best thing for acute orthopedic injuries (Marquez-Lara, 2016). Another example of this shift in medical understanding is arthroscopic knee surgeries. Historically, the knee meniscus was considered a vestigial remnant that had no significant impact on knee biomechanics. Consequently, thousands of patients underwent total or near-total removal of their knee meniscus. However, today, the decision to remove the knee meniscus is carefully considered because it can accelerate cartilage damage and result in the premature need for a knee replacement (Simonetta, 2023).

The Problem with Pain

Introducing Percutaneous Hydrotomy and Dr. Bernard Guez

Bernard Guez, a French general practitioner, is a multifaceted expert in the fields of regenerative medicine, aesthetics, mesotherapy and geriatrics. He developed a revolutionary regenerative medical technique called percutaneous hydrotomy, which employs physiologic saline (water), vitamins, minerals, and medications to treat chronic pain. This innovative technique can help you increase function and decrease pain, potentially avoiding surgery in many cases. Physiologic saline is a solution that closely matches the concentration of water and salts found in the human body.

One might wonder: Why isn't percutaneous hydrotomy widely known? One reason is that it's predominantly practiced and taught in French-speaking Europe. Dr. Guez has performed more than 400,000 procedures and has trained hundreds of healthcare practitioners from more than twenty-five countries in the technique. Dr. Guez's book *Vaincre les Maladies Chroniques* (Beating Chronic Disease), written in French and published in 2021, serves as a comprehensive guide to percutaneous hydrotomy (Guez, 2021). The process has also been presented in many scientific meetings in Europe and the United States.

Percutaneous hydrotomy was invented by Dr. Guez through his extensive knowledge of regenerative medicine and his desire to offer chronic pain patients more effective treatments than those provided by traditional medical systems. He created percutaneous hydrotomy through the principles of allopathic and alternative medicine practices, such as regenerative medicine, mesotherapy, oligotherapy, and aesthetics. However, these practices are still considered fringe areas within medicine despite impressive research; mesotherapy, oligotherapy, and percutaneous hydrotomy are seldom reported in mainstream medical journals. After three decades, percutaneous hydrotomy has reached a healthy scientific adolescence with the creation of the International Society of Percutaneous Hydrotomy (ISPH).

Percutaneous hydrotomy is a therapeutic procedure that addresses chronic pain, based on a sound understanding of medicine and human physiology and supported by numerous studies. Most importantly, it's a safe regenerative injection therapy based on well-established medical techniques and has been performed successfully hundreds of thousands of times. Additionally, the injections are minimally painful due to the use of tiny mesotherapy needles and diluted local anesthesia (Guez, 2021).

What's the difference between mesotherapy and percutaneous hydrotomy? They both involve injections with tiny needles but differ in several key aspects. The main difference is that percutaneous hydrotomy utilizes a larger volume of water and many substances traditionally used in mesotherapy, such as anti-inflammatories, vitamins, minerals, local anesthetics, and other compounds. Mesotherapy is better known as a cosmetic procedure, yet its original purpose was to treat chronic pain. For some indications, such as a frozen shoulder, the technique is the same for both treatments. However, in treating back pain, percutaneous hydrotomy utilizes a much larger volume of fluid to promote the dilution of pain chemicals, medications, and vitamins and has a longer residence time in the subcutaneous tissues, which will be explained in chapter 5.

The goal of percutaneous hydrotomy is to treat the root cause of the disease. By breaking the pain cycle and promoting natural healing, it addresses one of the most significant disabilities in modern times. Percutaneous hydrotomy is well designed to restore function and provide relief from various chronic ailments:

The Problem with Pain

- Migraines, fatigue, sinus problems, vertigo, and TMJ
- Back, neck, and knee pains, hip problems, and sciatica
- Frozen shoulder, bursitis, tendinitis, and rotator cuff issues
- Ankle arthritis, sprained or weak ankles, bunions, and other foot ailments
- Chronic allergies, Crohn's disease, and irritable bowel syndrome (IBS)

Dr. Bernard Guez's development of percutaneous hydrotomy was a culmination of years of experience and an understanding of well-established medical techniques in regenerative medicine, mesotherapy, oligotherapy, hypodermoclysis, and tumescent anesthesia. These techniques, backed by extensive medical research and a strong safety record, played a crucial role in its creation.

For example, hypodermoclysis is a medical technique that infuses fluids into the subcutaneous tissue (the layer of skin just below the dermis). Hypodermoclysis has been used for hydration for centuries in children and geriatric patients due to its ease of administration. Tumescent anesthesia, developed by dermatologist Dr. Jeffrey Klein, is now the gold standard in plastic surgery, involving the injection of large volumes of diluted local anesthesia into the subcutaneous tissue. As for mesotherapy, it's based on the concept that administering medications in the superficial skin layer, which provides longer pharmacological action in the painful area, requires lower doses compared to intramuscular injections, bypasses the digestive system, and achieves fewer side effects compared to systemic administration. Even for vaccines, intradermal injections have demonstrated a superior antibody response with lower doses (Pitzurra, 1981).

Stopping Pain

Dr. Michel Pistor is widely recognized as the father of mesotherapy. He developed the technique in the 1950s, has gained international recognition from the French Academy of Medicine since 2005, and is now taught in universities worldwide. Even though mesotherapy is predominantly known for cosmetic use, it was originally developed to treat pain, vascular conditions, and sports injuries. It's a minimally invasive medical procedure where a solution of medications and other products are injected below the skin's dermis layer using tiny needles for the treatment of specific conditions (Mammucari, 2020). The practice of mesotherapy varies significantly in regulation and acceptance from country to country.

It was in the 1980s that the concept of percutaneous hydrotomy was conceived through discussions with Drs. Guez and Pistor. Both were passionate about the future of mesotherapy, and they discussed the potential of applying mesotherapy principles and water to treat individuals with chronic pain. They expanded mesotherapy's principles to create what they then initially called mesotherapy and hydration and surface mesotherapy. After fifteen years of observation and refinement, Dr. Guez decided to introduce the term "percutaneous hydrotomy" within medical circles. Through empirical observation and experience, Guez and Pistor treated patients with large volumes of saline, local anesthetics, minerals, anti-inflammatories, vasodilators, and chelating agents, finding it particularly beneficial for patients with chronic back pain. Vasodilators are medications that cause dilation of blood vessels and serve to increase drug penetration into the affected area. Chelating agents are chemical compounds that bind to metal ions. We'll learn more about this in Chapter 5.

The essential message of percutaneous hydrotomy and other regenerative techniques is that chronic pain doesn't have to be endured. By embracing the principles of percutaneous hydrotomy, you can harness your body's inherent self-healing capacities and maintain good health. Many people have inquired about the nature of percutaneous hydrotomy and how it differs from allopathic (conventional) medicine, which often treats symptoms as causes and mislabels them as diseases. While the questions might appear simple, humans are intricate and complex beings, each unique in their healing journey. This approach instills the confidence to understand that our bodies are designed to heal themselves, and healing is an internal process.

In other words, healing is an inside job.

Dr. Edwards's Journey into Percutaneous Hydrotomy

My introduction into percutaneous hydrotomy began fortuitously when I met Sam Calavitta, a world-renowned athletic coach also known as Coach Cal. It seemed like serendipitous fate or chance had brought Coach Cal and me together. We both grew up in the small desert town of Victorville, California, and attended the same church and schools. One day, Coach Cal sought my opinion on a medical procedure being practiced in France that utilized water's power to heal musculoskeletal injuries.

"Hey Doc." Coach Cal's voice on the phone was filled with enthusiasm. "I want to send a couple of my athletes to France to get this new percutaneous hydrotomy procedure. What do you think?" At that moment my imagination spun into motion. As a medical doctor, I deduced that percutaneous meant through the skin and hydrotomy had something to do with water; I imagined it must be related to injecting water into the skin. Water's potential healing abilities have been well researched (Altman, 2016; Pollack, 2012; Saltzman 2017; Previtali 2021; Gao, 2019; Acosto-Olivo, 2020; Gazendam 2021; Vora, 2012).

Stopping Pain

Coach Cal is a brilliant man and a numbers-oriented guy. Trained as a mathematician and a former aerospace engineer, he excelled as an educator and was awarded the prestigious Siemens award for being one of the best calculus teachers in the United States with nearly every one of his students acing the AP calculus exam every year (Calavitta, 2010). His teaching philosophy developed from years competing as a wrestler and in Ironman Triathlons. He is also the father of nine children; naturally, they all are very good at math.

Coach Cal said, "I was hoping you could do this procedure, so my athletes won't have to go to France." I was curious and intrigued about percutaneous hydrotomy because, as an anesthesiologist, I have injected plenty of medicines below the skin. I wanted to know more. I promised Coach Cal that I would review the procedure and get back to him.

A few weeks later, I asked Coach Cal how he became interested in the technique. He explained that he was in contact with a medical doctor who introduced him to Quinton marine water. Intrigued by marine water therapy, Cal spent several months researching and discovered René Quinton, who administered subcutaneous purified marine water to thousands of children suffering from kwashiorkor, a malnutrition disease.

One of Coach Cal's athletes, Olympic wrestler Bo Nickal, was experiencing back pain due to a protruding herniated disc measuring 11 mm in his lumbar spine. Bo had tried every conventional medical modality, including physical therapy, medications, and epidural steroid injections, but he was still struggling. With an upcoming match against another Olympic athlete, David Taylor, who later won a gold medal in the 2021 Tokyo Olympics, it became apparent that Bo Nickal needed to try this procedure before he underwent spine surgery. As a result, he booked a flight to France.

The Problem with Pain

Cal's intuition is often proved to be correct. A few weeks before Bo's trip, he spoke to me about a physician named Dr. Bernard Guez, who performs percutaneous hydrotomy procedures in Nice, France. All Coach Cal knew was that it involved using water to heal injuries and had a remarkable success rate.

There are only two things a person needs to say to me to spark my interest—something about healing and anything about France. Growing up, I had a strong desire to experience living outside the United States, so I chose to complete a year of my medical training in Lyon, France. At the University of Claude Bernard, I learned many concepts not typically taught in US medical schools.

One such concept is the French term *terrain*, derived from the Latin word *terra*, meaning earth. To the French, terrain not only refers to the health of the soil, where plants and animals grow, but also carries a deeper meaning, signifying the overall health of the Earth. French culture places a strong emphasis on nurturing both the environment and the human body, particularly the water and cells that compose our bodies. Just like the soil, our bodies are composed of countless cells, and these cells constitute our terrain. The French are among the world's longest-living people. Perhaps more importantly, they maintain high functionality well into their later years (Prioux, 2012). It's not uncommon to see individuals in their seventies engaging in forty-kilometer hikes. The French embrace alternative, complementary, and Western healing methods and know that treating their bodies like the earth leads to good health and longevity.

Delving deeper into percutaneous hydrotomy, I discovered its roots in the French ideas of mesotherapy and its application in treating arthritis and other ailments (Guez, 2019). As an anesthesiologist, the procedure appeared relatively straightforward. I read and

Stopping Pain

watched every research article and video available on the website at www.percutaneoushydrotomy.net.

One particularly notable study from Italy treated patients with calcific tendinitis of the shoulder, or frozen shoulder, which is characterized by pain and limited range of motion, significantly affecting one's quality of life. The Italian doctors administered multiple subcutaneous injections of saline, magnesium, local anesthetics, and a chelating agent called ethylenediaminetetraacetic acid (EDTA) over the painful areas over six weeks (Cachio, 2009). The results were compelling, with nearly every patient experiencing a reduction in pain and a gain in function. Before-and-after X-rays show the disappearance of the calcium in the tendons (Cachio, 2009). As a medical doctor, I understand that there are many therapies for frozen shoulder, but most were not taught about this method.

The possibilities of percutaneous hydrotomy seemed promising. Although I was still skeptical, I wondered if percutaneous hydrotomy could work for my elbow arthritis, which was preventing me from playing my favorite sport, tennis. I'd been experiencing elbow pain for months and had it evaluated by an orthopedic surgeon who injected it with a cortisone shot, which did nothing. My curiosity abounded; I then embarked on the ultimate scientific experiment and opted to try the procedure on myself. In my clinic, I set everything I needed on the table and made the hydrotomy solution. First, I injected the local anesthetic tumescent in my elbow and then subcutaneously injected the area of pain with a mixture of saline, vitamins, and anti-inflammatories. Afterward, I thought, "I hope there's something to this, because there is a lot of fluid in there." Within a couple of hours, the soreness and swelling subsided. The following morning, my elbow felt

The Problem with Pain

much better. It was functional, and both the pain and the range of motion in my elbow had improved. I swung my tennis racket without pain, which I'd not been able to do before the treatment. I remember asking myself, "What kind of magic is this?" Questions were swimming through my head, particularly about its potential to treat people with back pain, arthritis, and even athletes. What else did percutaneous hydrotomy treat?

Excitedly, I called Coach Cal to share the good news about how the procedure seemed to work. His Olympic wrestler, Bo Nickal, was still in need of relief from his back pain. The plan was now for me to go to France to receive proper training in the procedure and then treat Bo.

Motivated to learn as much as possible, I contacted the International Society of Percutaneous Hydrotomy in France and inquired about their upcoming 2020 course. Unfortunately, they informed me that the course was "complet" and that I would have to wait until the following year. Disappointed, I shared this news with Coach Cal, and he began arranging Bo's travel to France to undergo the treatment.

However, a few days later, I received an email from Dr. Guez himself. He informed me that he could accommodate me in the upcoming course, which also happened to be his last one, as he was preparing for retirement from clinical practice. Thrilled by the opportunity, I signed up for the course and booked my flights to France.

However, a new challenge arose—the French borders were closed to American travelers due to the COVID-19 pandemic. To gain entry, I needed to show an exemption letter from the International Society of Percutaneous Hydrotomy, confirming my status as a "foreign talent" attending a medical meeting. Fortunately, Dr. Guez provided me with the necessary letter. I flew to France, and I had the paperwork to clear French customs and proceed with my plans.

Stepping onto French soil felt invigorating. The next morning, I woke up and relished a fresh baked croissant and a café au lait. I walked to the hotel where the course was being held; it was situated in the heart of Nice, on the Promenade d'Anglais. At the hotel, Dr. Guez warmly greeted me, seemingly surprised by my fluent French. He expressed his delight that I was at the course and promptly began the lectures.

Dr. Guez began with the history and the theory behind percutaneous hydrotomy. He first reviewed René Quinton's work in the 1900s based on Dr. Michel Pistor's development of mesotherapy in 1952. Dr. Guez explained how percutaneous hydrotomy was focused on treating the biological terrain, or the body's environment or ecosystem, and how everything is interconnected by the five units of competence which are the fundamental parts of understanding percutaneous hydrotomy (see Chapter 5). The lectures stretched well into the evening, and as the jet lag ensued, it became challenging to stay focused. After a week of lectures absorbing knowledge about percutaneous hydrotomy, it was time to see it performed in the clinic.

I had the opportunity to observe and participate in percutaneous hydrotomy treatments at Dr. Guez's clinic in Nice, France. The clinic is situated in the heart of Nice, has three exam rooms, an office, and a mixing room. I was there with three others, two nurses and another physician. Dr. Guez is not your typical French doctor. He starts very early in the morning and sees thirty to fifty patients daily, often until late evening, barely pausing for lunch. During my training, I witnessed numerous successful percutaneous hydrotomy treatments for various medical conditions. Dr. Guez possesses an

The Problem with Pain

unwavering curiosity; he wants to understand the thought processes of individuals. In the middle of the injections, he often engages the students in discussion about the root causes of a patient's chronic disease and then explains how percutaneous hydrotomy can help. He emphasizes the aim of alleviating the patients' pain and reducing their dependence on medications. It was clear that percutaneous hydrotomy can potentially help people by channeling the body's energies toward healing. My experience in medicine has taught me that healing cannot take place without the movement of energy.

In the clinic, we encountered men, women, and children with various chronic diseases, including arthritis, hand contractures, migraines, severe allergies, and neck and back pain, among others. I was shown how to treat many of these chronic diseases using a combination of physiologic saline, vitamins, anti-inflammatories, and local anesthetics. As I was leaving the clinic, I couldn't help but ask Dr. Guez why he opened a spot for me in the course. With a smile, he revealed that I was the first American medical doctor interested in being trained in percutaneous hydrotomy.

Walking in the *vieux ville*, or old city, of Nice, I realized the start of something important. Throughout my career in sports medicine, I have worked with professional and amateur athletes in football, cycling, running, UFC mixed martial arts combat, motocross, and tennis. Additionally, I have served as a doctor for the Dakar Rally, professional cycling races, and marathons. I was anxious and hopeful about how percutaneous hydrotomy would help my patients, and I could see its potential, especially for athletes who suffer back pain.

Upon my return to the United States, Coach Cal and Bo Nickal traveled to my clinic. I performed the percutaneous hydrotomy procedure on Bo's back, and he soon reported good pain relief and resumed his normal activities. He started training again two weeks later and eventually returned to competition, pain free. Since the treatment, Bo Nickal has become one of the hottest prospects in the UFC, the premier mixed martial arts organization. He has an exceptional career ahead of him. I have since treated many patients like Bo and have become confident that percutaneous hydrotomy can help many people. It is not a panacea, or even a miracle, but it does decrease pain, restore function, and increase movement. Most importantly, it does all this without toxic medications; this is what regenerative medicine does.

The following year, I returned to Nice for the annual meeting of the International Society of Percutaneous Hydrotomy. I had the privilege of giving a case presentation (in French) about how percutaneous hydrotomy successfully treated the shoulder of a prominent UFC fighter named T.J. Dillashaw. I presented a series of slides showing how it helped T.J.'s shoulder injury improve in six weeks and how it contributed to him winning his comeback fight. The presentation was well received, and I answered many questions regarding the practice of percutaneous hydrotomy in the United States.

A few days later, I rendezvoused with Dr. Guez in a hotel on the Promenade des Anglais. I could sense both the excitement and the trepidation in his eyes. By this point, we knew each other well. Dr. Guez's life mission revolved around helping as many patients as possible through percutaneous hydrotomy. His book, *Vaincre les Maladies Chroniques* (Beating Chronic Disease), had garnered significant success in France, but the book needed to be written in English so the rest of the world could learn about percutaneous hydrotomy. I knew I could translate the book from French to English. I had already done this with my other book, *The Science of the Marathon* (Billat, 2021). But the new book needed to

The Problem with Pain

accomplish something greater. It needed to show that Dr. Guez is the authority in this area of medicine, that the procedure is safe, and that it helps patients. Percutaneous hydrotomy is Dr. Guez's life work, something he's been developing for over thirty years. As the first American to learn this practice, it seemed only natural for me to write the book. We agreed that I would write the book about percutaneous hydrotomy in English and give the world another tool to battle chronic pain.

Giving Patients New Hope to Transform Chronic Pain

Percutaneous hydrotomy takes a complementary approach—encompassing the mind, body, and spirit to treat the root cause of diseases. A broader view of human well-being doesn't isolate particular systems but recognizes that all systems are interrelated. The current medical paradigm commits an error when trying to isolate and treat only the pain. The result is often worse, which is why the human organism is a complex system.

The Nobel laureate in medicine, Albert Szent-Györgyi, highlighted that in every culture and every medical tradition before ours, healing was accomplished by moving energy (Györgyi, 1972). Three decades ago, anyone offering any form of alternative medicine was going out on a limb, scientifically speaking. Since then, scientific literature has seen an explosion of studies on alternative healing methods (Simon, 1999). Alternative medicine gained a rite of passage into Western medicine in 1992 when the National Institutes of Health (NIH) established the office of alternative medicine, later renamed the National Center for Complementary and Integrative Health. Dr. Jay Bhattacharya is the current NIH director and he has a willingness to consider unconventional ideas that are supported by science (personal communication, 2022).

Stopping Pain

This new convention conveys a different normative message. "Alternative medicine" might suggest a departure from the high road of official medicine, whereas "complementary medicine" implies that biomedicine can benefit by integrating with other medical traditions. Healthcare providers of all types stand to benefit through cooperation rather than competing against one another. In 2007, Dr. Mehmet Oz, one of America's foremost physicians and then director of the Cardiovascular Institute at Columbia University, stated on *The Oprah Winfrey Show* that one of the next frontiers is energy medicine. It's ironic that Dr. Oz is currently President Donald Trump's administrator of the Centers for Medicare and Medicaid Services (CMS), which provides coverage provides health coverage to more than 160 million through Medicare, Medicaid, the Children's Health Insurance Program, as well as working with the newly appointed HHS director, Robert F. Kennedy Jr. Many younger healthcare providers recognize that the future of alternative and complementary medicine is bright.

Healing is truly a multipronged process and most healthcare providers focus on one thing: the body. But the root cause of pain always involves the mind, body, and spirit; for example, knee pain can result from a poor back position or weak hips, but without an improvement in function, corrective rehabilitation is nearly impossible. Then the pain becomes ingrained in our minds and becomes a repetitive cycle, often leading to depression. This, in combination with the lack of support from family and from healing institutions, eventually breaks our spirit.

With this book, you're one step closer to regaining function and moving toward a pain-free body! This book highlights many stories of patients who have been taking medications for ten or twenty years, but they never recover; these patients carry their pain with no

The Problem with Pain

prospect of relief—until now. We aim to offer hope by presenting an innovative vision of medicine throughout the world of percutaneous hydrotomy. By taking advantage of the extraordinary regenerative powers of our bodies, percutaneous hydrotomy provides the fundamental elements so that the cells and organs can be nourished, strengthened, and repaired. This technique finally gives us a clear, practical, mechanical answer to chronic pain. Where conventional medicine only masks the pain, percutaneous hydrotomy offers a therapeutic alternative that targets the causes of the disease and not just the symptoms.

The International Society of Percutaneous Hydrotomy has dedicated itself to the development of this technique for over twenty years and has trained hundreds of healthcare providers. The society's website, www.percutaneoushydrotomy.net, attracts hundreds of thousands of unique visitors each year. This book will present the problems with modern medicine's approach to pain management and why percutaneous hydrotomy is a safe and effective method for treating chronic diseases. Chapter 9 presents numerous patient testimonials of how it has improved their quality of life.

In the upcoming chapters, we will explore why chronic disease is so prevalent in modern society, provide a comprehensive understanding of the root cause of an injury, and demonstrate the importance of regenerative medicine and percutaneous hydrotomy in addressing these issues.

CHAPTER 2

Medicine in a Changing World

For many, chronic diseases are a part of their daily lives, but they needn't be. According to the Merriam-Webster dictionary, the term *chronic* means "continuing or occurring again and again for a long time." Using this simpler view, we would exclude something like a broken leg as a chronic condition but include recurring lower back pain or migraine headaches.

The phrase "chronic disease" is a term often used in discussions between patients and healthcare providers, as well as among friends and family, academic literature, and policy discussions. Popular internet sources and governmental agencies use "chronic disease" or "chronic condition" to mean slightly different things. For instance, there exists considerable variation in the duration of a condition required for it to be classified as chronic. The most widely accepted definition of a chronic injury is one that has not healed in six weeks (Carlson, 2011).

Rather than adhering to a specific list of diseases and time frames, we advocate for a more straightforward approach. A chronic

Medicine in a Changing World

disease consists of multiple complex causal risk factors, a long development period for which there may or may not be symptoms, and associated functional impairment or disability (Bernell, 2021). It's a prolonged illness, often associated with other health complications (Zelaya, 2019). Chronic diseases are costly and taxing for patients and their caregivers. We now talk about "years lived with a disability" when speaking of chronic diseases, such as pain, depression, and anxiety.

Back pain has been called "the evil of the century." Inexplicably, modern medicine only partially responds to this disease. Low back and neck pain resulting from arthritis is the single greatest cause of disability and chronic pain, affecting approximately 600 million people worldwide. Astonishingly, the incidence of back pain has nearly tripled over the past forty years (Ferreira, 2021). People know something's wrong, and back pain is the tip of the iceberg of what's happening today.

Back pain is the most prevalent source of pain and complex due to its multifaceted nature involving biological, psychological, and social components (Mills, 2019). According to a CDC Data Brief in 2020, more than 20 percent of US adults had chronic pain, and 7.4 percent of adults had chronic pain that significantly limited life or work activities (Zelaya, 2019). Furthermore, in 2019, the National Health Interview survey found that nearly 59 percent of adults reported experiencing pain on a regular basis in the past three months, with 39 percent reporting back pain (Ferreira, 2021).

Due to the difficulties in treating the root cause of chronic low back pain, an overreliance on opioid pain medications often develops, increasing the risk of overdose and death (Mauck, 2023). It's worth noting that 50 percent of European workers claim they have suffered from back pain in the last twelve months. In France, a report from the National Agency for the Safety of Medicines and Health Products highlighted that nearly 20 million French people (about 30 percent of the adult population) suffer from chronic pain and are resistant to conventional analgesic treatments (Guez, 2021). Many people continue to suffer for most of their natural lives, with little chance of recovery. According to the World Health Organization (WHO), the number of people living with low back pain is predicted to increase substantially over the coming decades, driven largely by population expansion, poor physical condition, and aging (Vos, 2016).

Migraine headaches represent another major cause of chronic pain, leading to serious disruptions in daily life. Why migraines are so prevalent remains unclear. The Global Burden of Disease Study reaffirmed that 1.9 billion people were affected by recurrent tension-type headaches and are often forced to take medications indefinitely (Vos, 2016).

Where does current medicine stand in the face of this enormous problem? Pain is the number one reason people seek healthcare providers. The problem is that most patients prefer prescription analgesic medications to address their chronic pain. Likewise, the healthcare providers prefer to prescribe these medications, which do nothing to cure the disease. Pain patients are the largest consumers of anti-inflammatories and antidepressants. Why is this the case? Despite these treatments, their pain is always present, and worse, they are chained in a vicious cycle of constantly taking medications.

A striking example of this issue is when the modern medical system refuses to satisfactorily address the problem. Western physicians are aware of the limitations in effectively treating chronic diseases (Brunner-La Roca, 2016). The initial response often involves prescribing medications while disregarding the role of emotions or the resulting depression from being unable to maintain an active life. Rarely do we ask about the person's history of psychological trauma. One fundamental problem is that Western medicine primarily views chronic diseases solely as a biological problem, when it's an embodiment of the mind, body, and spirit. A well-known physician, Dr. Gabor Maté, eloquently states that chronic illness is the body's expression of experiences, beliefs, and lifelong patterns of relations to self and the world (Maté, 2022). The word *healing* means wholeness, and when we become whole, we can reconnect with ourselves and elevate our consciousness. Percutaneous hydrotomy treats the body as a complex system rather than a paint-by-numbers checklist.

Clinical Case: Mr. P., fifty-five years old

Chronic Back Pain

My lower back pain started about twenty-five years ago while working at my construction job. I did nothing about it for eight to ten years. Then it started affecting my life and the doctor scheduled an MRI, which showed the expected results of degenerative disc disease at L3 to S1 (four levels), facet joint damage, and foraminal narrowing. I managed my back pain with weight loss, stretching, and an occasional cortisone shot. Three months ago, my back became so painful I had to seek treatment. They offered me surgery, but this wasn't an option in my mind. My trainer told me about the percutaneous hydrotomy treatment for my back, which sounded like something that could help with my back pain. I went to Dr. Edwards's clinic, and we did the procedure.

Stopping Pain

> The next morning, I was amazed. I could touch my toes, and my back was no longer in excruciating pain. After a week, I tried to play golf to test if my back would hold up. In the past, I always had more back pain after playing golf. My back was fine. It has been ten weeks since I had the treatment, and my back is pain free.

Medicine has devolved into a standardized, paint-by-numbers approach, meaning healthcare providers emphasize a checklist to manage diseases rather than individualizing care. While this sometimes works for diseases of the heart and lungs, it's quite another to say it helps in chronic diseases like migraines and back pain. Chronic pain patients are seeking pain relief and a return to normalcy, which can be achieved through individualized care, talking with the patient, regular visits, assessing the patient's personal and family history, putting together the information from medical tests, and relying on the intuition of both the patient and healthcare provider.

Most medications are unjustified or unnecessary. Pharmaceutical companies have created direct-to-consumer advertising strategies costing billions of dollars to maximize profits. The result is increased drug prices and consumption of medications. The number of Americans taking multiple medications nearly doubled from 2000 to 2012 from 8 to 15 percent. With nearly half of adults over the age of sixty-five taking five or more medications, we're seeing a sharp rise in adverse drug events, leading to millions of unnecessary hospitalizations (Brownlee, 2008). Take rheumatoid arthritis as an example. It affects over 350 million worldwide, and the treatments offered (drugs, physiotherapy, injections, and operations) rarely change anything. Despite treatment, one study found that almost 75 percent of rheumatoid patients are dissatisfied with their treatments (Radawski, 2019).

What can be done? Now, more than ever, is the time to rethink our approach to medicine. Ideally, we need medical techniques that address the root cause of diseases and intervene directly within the origin of the ailment. Healthcare providers should focus on listening to patients and stop masking symptoms with chemicals. This pain is experienced in the flesh, and we must use it as a therapeutic guide. When experiencing pain, we must consider treating the body's fundamental unit—our cells.

If you're suffering from chronic disease, take a moment to think about today's world and how today's pain is different. Where does chronic disease originate? These are undoubtedly open-ended questions, but dramatic changes in socioeconomic status, population growth, and agriculture have culminated in imbalances in our bodies (Heying, 2021). Nearly everyone's lifestyle has veered from the natural order of human development. Our evolution is for a world that hasn't existed for hundreds of years; movement as a necessity for survival is a relic of the past. In the 1900s, manual laborers outnumbered skilled workers, but by the 1980s, the reverse was true (Heying, 2021). These transformations have manifested too rapidly, not giving our bodies time to strengthen and protect themselves. For example, antibiotics can have unintended consequences for the good bacteria in our intestines. Antibiotics are designed to kill all bacteria and don't distinguish between good and harmful bacteria. Disruption of our good bacteria can result in diarrhea, malabsorption of vitamins and diminished immune function.

Our bodies are designed for adaptation, but this blink in the evolutionary lens is far too brief for natural selection to have updated the arrangement. These mutations influence the anatomy of our intestinal microbiota and, thus, the adaptation of our immune system. Moreover, psycho-emotional factors such as stress contribute to the weakening of our immune defenses.

Industrialization has radically shifted our environment and is marked by technological advances in medicine, religion, education, and work. Visionary entrepreneurs like Jeff Bezos and Elon Musk are sending tourists to space in commercial rocket ships. It's now commonplace to work from home with smartphones and computers; television and the internet are endless; population growth has exploded. In the past two decades, some of the most substantial changes are the genome, quantum science, drugs, pharmaceuticals, food science, and climate science. Many of these have contributed significantly to humans living longer—just fifty years ago, we were surviving into our seventies; today, we are surviving into our eighties and beyond. However, increased longevity and prosperity bring more chronic diseases. While humanity is inarguably better in many ways (e.g., reduction in global poverty), it has deteriorated in others (e.g., heightened risk of nuclear war).

We've adapted to the industrial and postindustrial world with software designed for living in the wild. We've forgotten that we're completely connected to nature. Humans have become so technologically advanced in recent decades that we now have the power to destroy both the world and our health.

The costs of adapting to an environment where our bodies didn't evolve are observable in today's chronic diseases. For example, nearly one-third of the global working population is engaged in night shift work, especially healthcare workers (Shi, 2022). Research has highlighted that night shift work disrupts circadian rhythms, increases sleep disturbances, and causes other behavioral changes,

Medicine in a Changing World

leading to an increased risk of chronic diseases, mental disorders, cognition impairment, and mortality in nurses (Shi, 2022). The World Health Organization's International Agency for Research on Cancer concludes that shift work is likely carcinogenic for humans (Erren, 2019).

We have more chronic diseases than at any time in history (Holman, 2020). It's estimated that half of sixty-five-year-olds can't get up from the floor with one or two hands (Kubitza, 2022)—it's worth pausing for a moment to let that sink in. We've surrendered to living with chronic diseases like arthritis, headaches, cardiovascular disease, gastrointestinal diseases, and cancer. Despite the last three American presidents, Obama, Trump, and Biden, having implemented policies to combat chronic diseases, nothing seems to change. Even billionaire entrepreneurs like Bill Gates and Elon Musk suffer from chronic diseases despite their vast resources.

But why? One reason is that we've polluted many resources essential to life—our agriculture, air, and water. The chemicals we employ in various industries are turning up in our lakes, rivers, and oceans. A stark example is California, which dumps millions of gallons of wastewater into the Pacific Ocean daily (SeaWeb, 2008). Our drinking water is polluted and laden with chemicals; coal, oil, and diesel are burned into the atmosphere; we breathe toxic levels of nitrogen oxide and sulfur dioxide, affecting every cell in our bodies; technology has introduced electromagnetic radiation everywhere. All this has affected our bodies in ways never imagined. Normally, our immune systems keep us safe from microbes and certain foods, but with thousands of artificial chemicals in our food and air, our immune systems remain in a heightened state of emergency that depletes our energy and our life force (Kau, 2011).

Meanwhile, we're always teetering on the edge of the fight-or-flight response. Indeed, this heightened state is among nature's most brilliant achievements, but it was never intended to cope with the perpetual stressors we face today: work-related stress, financial pressures, relationship challenges, technology overload, health concerns, time management, social pressures, environmental factors, and personal expectations. Our biological systems are ill-equipped to navigate these unfamiliar and constant stressors; our systems aren't adapted to biologically unfamiliar environments.

Our digestive tracts are perfectly designed to extract minerals and nutrients from our diets and release these nutrients into our bloodstream, from which they then find their way into the specific cells that require them. Over the last sixty years, intensive farming practices have depleted many trace minerals from the food we eat. Millions of people are now deficient in essential minerals, giving rise to obesity and chronic diseases through a phenomenon known as hidden hunger. This, combined with the overuse of refined salts, contributes to our chronic diseases (Ibeanu, 2020).

Farm animals are routinely given antibiotics not to treat an illness, but rather to increase their weight and therefore the farmer's profits. Animals are raised on antibiotics, producing meat that lowers our immune defenses by disrupting intestinal microbiota. Modified wheat and dairy also negatively affect our intestines. Radiation from nonnative electromagnetic waves (e.g., smartphones, relay antennas, 4G, 5G, Wi-Fi, microwaves) creates fields that disturb human biological tissues, and their long-term effects are poorly understood (Becker, 1998; Muscat, 2000). An inefficiency of our natural immune system increases our susceptibility to viruses, bacteria, allergies, autoimmune diseases, and even cancers. This unstable environment promotes the development of chronic diseases, and an explosion of chronic diseases is predictable within the next ten years (Ansah, 2023).

The Malady of Modern Medicine

The human body is complex, and reductionist thinking is harming us. One of the challenges with modern medicine lies in the reductionist approach, which purports that complex problems can be solved by breaking them down into smaller parts. This approach inevitably reduces complex behaviors to a simple set of variables with the goal of identifying a cause and an effect. While breaking complex phenomena into parts is a valuable scientific method, there are certain situations, especially in medicine, where the approach doesn't work. Complex systems are by there nature complex; we cannot heal the human body using machines with codes and parts.

Consider the example of strep throat, a bacterial infection commonly treated with antibiotics. While some individuals may experience improvement after taking antibiotics, many others do not. The high number of individuals who continue to suffer from strep throat raises questions about the effectiveness of antibiotics as a stand-alone treatment. This highlights the limitations of reductionism as it relates to the complexity of human health (Heying, 2022). Another common example is reducing calories to lose weight. This approach fails to consider the complexity of additional calories, whether the calories derive from carbohydrate versus protein versus fat, or whether they derive from whole versus highly processed foods.

An evolutionary example of reductionist thinking is the addition of fluoride to our drinking water. While the intention was to reduce dental disease, it's important to consider the unintended consequences. The fluoride added to drinking water is not identical to the fluoride found in nature. If fluoride is intended for our dental health, why do we need it everywhere in our body? Fluoride is toxic to the nervous systems of developing children by competing with iodine. It harms our brains and our thyroid glands. In the case of fish, exposure to fluoride in rivers causes salmon to lose their ability to navigate to native streams and therefore hinders reproduction (SeaWeb, 2008).

Modern medicine has been masking the symptoms of diseases with pharmaceuticals rather than treating the cause; even worse, the response to medication side effects is to take more medicines to counteract the side effects of those other medicines. Pharmaceutical companies have taken advantage of this situation by creating numerous drugs used in our daily lives. New drug production is the focus of pharmaceutical companies; they allocate vast sums of money to research with the hope of beneficial financial returns. Pharmaceutical companies excel in creating voluminous documents, adapting perfectly to the requests of government health authorities. These expensive studies always find their way into the FDA-approved drug's ultimate cost, and in the end, it's the patient who pays. Market forces push for profits, leading to less time for interaction between the patient and the healthcare provider.

The Rise and Fall of Vioxx: An American Tragedy

Pharmaceutical companies don't always have your best interests at heart. An illustrative case is that of Merck, who produced a nonsteroidal anti-inflammatory drug (NSAID) called Vioxx to treat patients with arthritis. Vioxx is in a class of anti-inflammatories

Medicine in a Changing World

called COX-2 inhibitors, which were heavily touted as having fewer side effects than older NSAIDs. Merck released Vioxx to the public in May 1999, and it gained widespread use among healthcare providers treating arthritis and other chronic diseases.

The *New England Journal of Medicine* (*NEJM*) published an article on November 23, 2000, in which the authors concluded Vioxx had a safety advantage over an older drug, naproxen, because it caused fewer serious stomach complications. However, four years later, on September 30, 2004, Merck voluntarily pulled Vioxx off the market after completing a study showing that it doubled the risk of heart attacks and strokes. Three weeks later, the FDA finally pulled Vioxx off the market after a seventeen-year-old girl died of a stroke days after taking it. It was the largest drug recall in history. Eighty million people worldwide had taken the drug over the previous five years. Patients were taking Vioxx to relieve their aches and pains from arthritis while unknowingly doubling their risk of heart attacks and strokes.

Merck knew Vioxx caused heart attacks and strokes years before withdrawing the drug. The malfeasance doesn't end there. In his book, *Sickening: How Big Pharma Broke American Health Care and How We Can Repair It*, John Abramson, MD, states that Merck scientists distributed an email in March 2000 about the cardiovascular dangers of Vioxx. Merck researchers falsified the statistics by omitting heart attacks to avoid a statistical threshold. In addition, Dr. Scott Reuben, a professor of anesthesiology at Tufts University, published several studies on COX-2 inhibitors and was considered an authority on the subject. Later, he admitted that he never conducted the clinical trials he published in twenty-one journal articles about COX-2 inhibitors. Dr. Reuben had fabricated the data and overstated the analgesic effects of the drugs. *Scientific American* labeled Reuben the medical equivalent of Bernie Madoff.

Merck knew as early as 1996 that humans taking Vioxx were at greater risk of cardiovascular problems. Merck covered the effects of cardiovascular problems in the studies by giving patients daily aspirin. They failed the world by not being forthright about the risk of heart attack and stroke associated with Vioxx. The *NEJM* failed the world by not setting the record straight about the November 2000 Vioxx article. Even worse, the *NEJM* remained silent for over four years and never attempted to correct the Vioxx article. They only wrote a "letter of concern" a year after they took the drug off the market. The FDA failed the world by not informing healthcare providers about the cardiovascular risks of Vioxx. Furthermore, the FDA didn't stop Merck from buying nearly a million reprints of the incomplete and falsely reassuring *NEJM* article handed out to millions of healthcare providers. Merck had put more into its advertising campaign for Vioxx than any other drug in its history.

In the end, Vioxx was responsible for between 88,000 and 140,000 heart attacks from 1999 to 2004, killing 40,000 to 60,000 Americans. Merck paid over $5 billion to settle civil litigation and illegal marketing penalties, which was only a fraction of what they ultimately earned from the drug; Merck made over $11 billion from Vioxx during its four years on the market. The very sources healthcare providers rely on to inform their clinical decisions have become profit-driven rather than science-driven (Abramson, 2002; Prakash, 2007).

Medicine in a Changing World

The overconsumption of pain medicines is stifling—millions of boxes of them are sold annually in the United States (Leopoldino, 2019). Their long-term daily use can cause serious adverse effects, even death. For example, a quarter of the US population takes Tylenol each week (Brune, 2015), despite its limited effectiveness. Opioid-derived drugs like codeine, tramadol, and hydrocodone are prescribed with toxic doses of Tylenol, causing liver toxicity and sometimes necessitating liver transplants. One study affirmed that intentional and unintentional overdoses of Tylenol caused around 51 percent of cases of liver insufficiency (Larsen, 2005).

The situation in the United States is even more alarming regarding opioid-narcotic drugs. These drugs cloud thinking, lead to addiction, and, in the worst cases, result in death. According to CDC data, fatal drug overdose deaths in 2022 surpassed 110,000 (CDC, 2022). In 2023 it was hardly better, with 107,000 overdose deaths.

Drug reference books, once the size of a dictionary, have grown so large that they no longer fit in paper format and only exist digitally. New side effects have been discovered for old drugs, and laboratories have created newer drugs to counter them. But it turns out that these newfangled medications themselves carry additional side effects, creating a vicious cycle. Medication overload is the use of multiple medications for which the harm to the patient outweighs the benefit. Over the next ten years, it is predicted that there will be 4.6 million hospitalizations from medication overload.

According to the WHO, the future of medicine will be based on the quality of life. Indeed, if we force elderly patients to take medication to live normally for twenty-four hours and then start again every day until death, that patient's quality of life will be seriously affected. For lack of time, healthcare providers write prescriptions rather than listen to patients; without thinking, they prescribe analgesics for pain, antispasmodics for abdominal problems, and antihistamines for allergies without thoroughly considering the long-term consequences.

NSAIDs are commonly given to relieve chronic pain from osteoarthritis; however, they, too, can lead to heart and kidney failure, coronary diseases, heart attacks, and strokes (Hippisley-Cox, 2005; Lapeyre-Mestre 2013). High-dose corticosteroid injections can cause osteoporosis, tendon ruptures, and endocrine problems (Wong, 2020). Anti-seizure medications like gabapentin cause dizziness and drowsiness. Cyproterone, a testosterone-lowering drug for male contraception, can cause prostate cancer, brain cancer (meningiomas), and blood clots (Kuijpers, 2021). Long after patients have started these medications, we encounter daily restrictions on use, or a total withdrawal from the market, as with Vioxx.

Healthcare providers have a responsibility to critically assess the risk, benefits, and alternatives of medications and treatments for their patients. For example, medications for heartburn, such as proton pump inhibitors, have been found to cause dementia-related side effects (Haenisch, 2015; Ortiz-Guerrero, 2018). However, some patients become dependent on these medications and experience difficulties when trying to discontinue them. Many patients realize they can't live without these medications and take them for several years, incurring the side effects. Similarly, benzodiazepines are prescribed for sleep and anxiety, but they destroy sleep architecture. When patients stop taking them, the insomnia is even worse. Synthetic drugs have taken over the natural sleep facility, leaving people dependent on these medications (Garber, 2019). These examples are far from being exceptions.

Medicine in a Changing World

Healthcare providers are limiting themselves by temporarily stopping the symptoms but never treating the causes. The fundamental problem remains—painkillers don't treat the cause of the disease. As a result, we force patients to take increasingly higher doses, which become restrictive and dangerous. However, little remains in conventional medicine to treat chronic pain if these central analgesics are removed. We've observed the disappearance of inexpensive drugs that treat the cells, favoring modern drugs that don't treat the root cause of the lesion—but the pain will always remain by not addressing the cause. In addition, modern drugs are expensive, government health systems and insurances often deny coverage, and ultimately, the patient loses.

Clinical medicine is the wealth of information built by our predecessors over centuries. In the past, medical students focused on a traditional, highly scientific medical education with many intellectual achievements. Over the last century, the crux of medical practice has been based on scientific clinical observations using pathology, basic sciences, microbiology, biochemistry, physiology, pathophysiology, and anatomy. We learned about blood circulation in the 1800s through the groundbreaking work of pathologists who defined anatomy by dissecting cadavers. They stained biopsy specimens to understand what was happening at the microscopic level. A diagnosis is an artificial intellectual construct put together by close clinical observation and identifying patterns of symptoms looking for similarities in presentations between different patients. This is how we've come up with our taxonomy of disease. This way of thinking has been replaced with evidence-based medicine.

The Perils of Evidence-Based Medicine

The discussion about evidence-based medicine (EBM) and its implications is a complex and debated topic in the field of healthcare. Indeed, many advances have come about in emergent treatments such as acute heart attacks, stroke, and trauma, but double-blind studies and EBM don't result in the most beautiful medical discoveries. The general practitioner's office remains the best observation post for patient reactions following a therapeutic procedure.

1. **Challenges of Double-Blind Studies:** Conducting double-blind studies, which are a cornerstone of evidence-based medicine, can be impractical and ethically challenging in the context of general medical practice. In private practices where physicians have established relationships with their patients, it may be considered unethical to knowingly withhold potentially beneficial treatments for the sake of a study.
2. **Critique of Evidence-Based Medicine:** The rigid adherence to EBM guidelines may limit healthcare providers' ability to think critically, problem-solve, and practice clinical medicine effectively. This is seen as detrimental to patient care. It would be unthinkable that we can sacrifice the chances of curing our patients to compare the effect of a drug with a placebo.
3. **Totalitarian Influence:** EBM can have a totalitarian influence on medical practice, potentially displacing the doctor-patient relationship as the primary decision-making authority. Evidence-based medicine is a concept taught at universities and imposed in modern medicine. The current narrative is that all healthcare providers should practice EBM; however, it turns out not to be very scientific, and it's arguably more of a cult than of

science. Many healthcare practitioners have become dependent on EBM guidelines and have lost the ability to problem-solve, think critically, and practice clinical medicine. As a result, the patients are suffering the consequences.
4. **Agenda-Driven Actions:** The most gifted physicians have been forced out of practice and replaced by less skilled physicians and nurses. Such actions are unprecedented in the history of medicine and may have a detrimental impact on healthcare. When the only thing that matters is following guidelines, no thinking is necessary. We call this paint-by-numbers medicine.
5. **Influence of Pharmaceutical Companies:** EBM can be used to impose a form of medical dictatorship and grant undue power to corporate medicine and pharmaceutical companies, which have significant influence over universities and medical societies through financial contributions. This influence limits the exploration of treatments that may not be financially beneficial for these companies, particularly in the case of chronic pain conditions.
6. **Treatment of Chronic Conditions:** Treatment options for chronic conditions like back pain and depression often rely on older medical data and pharmaceuticals. These treatments often do not address the root causes of these conditions and may lead to patients needing to take medications for life (Amerling, 2021; Rai, 2012).

The claim that medicine is inadequate and that we must replace it with evidence-based medicine is highly questionable. We don't need a randomized-controlled trial (RCT) to know that fixing broken biology or physiology will have a favorable impact on outcomes. With the corporate takeover of medicine, most general practitioners and hospitalists are no longer accountable to their patients.

Instead, they are accountable to the insurance companies and the healthcare bureaucrats. The quality of medicine, personal enjoyment, creativity, and innovation that medicine once represented have vanished. Hospital-employed providers are constrained by the system, and if the hospital institutes guidelines, healthcare providers must adhere to them, or they will be replaced.

Getting Closer to Clinical Reality— Percutaneous Hydrotomy

Medicine is the art and the science of fostering physical, psychological, and spiritual health. In percutaneous hydrotomy, the healthcare provider is interested in the biological manifestations of the pain and the energy needed to heal the lesion. The Hippocratic oath says, "Do no harm." However, this is paradoxical because most treatments involve pain and suffering; therefore, we must constantly evaluate the risk-benefit ratio. Patients are seldom satisfied with doing nothing and reveal everything if we listen to them. The doctor-patient relationship is unique; it's the meeting of confidence and conscience. The patient's wishes are to stop the pain and to return to normal function without side effects. During the first meeting, the healthcare provider will create a file with the patient's medical and family history, the genesis of the illness, its duration, and the treatments undertaken. Then a treatment adapted to the patient will be proposed.

The recurring problem is polypharmacy, which is that the patient is taking too many medications. Most drugs are unjustified or unnecessary, particularly when considering the biological terrain, a concept that will be discussed in chapter 5. These drugs can be removed if we treat the disease's cause.

A nation concerned about the health and vitality of its population should react and invest more in this sector. In addition to

Medicine in a Changing World

the financial problems, there are also medical concerns regarding the long-term side effects of these drugs. Particularly for the elderly, who often take multiple medications, the side effects remain unknown. A world freed from polypharmacy would be of real added value.

The frontline general practitioner must become an artisan and work with their hands rather than a pen or a computer. This is called general interventional medicine (it already exists in cardiology and radiology). We aim to expand medications to treat chronic pain, allergies, hives, eczema, and much more. In these diseases that spread over time, the healthcare provider must find and treat the causes. Few things in life are as real as chronic pain; the answer is closer to a world with fewer drugs—this is precisely what percutaneous hydrotomy attempts to address.

In the practice of percutaneous hydrotomy, our focus extends beyond merely addressing symptoms and the names of the diseases. Instead, we prioritize the underlying biochemical problems of the pain that gives rise to pain and the injury. For example, osteoarthritis is primarily a biological phenomenon involving destructive degeneration, resulting in functional impotence. The goal of the consultation in percutaneous hydrotomy is to learn that the treatment will eliminate pain and medications. The patient is a wealth of information, and the truth always comes from them.

We have illustrated how medicine has changed, and the drastic results it has placed on society. Chronic pain remains a constant problem affecting the vitality of nations. In the next chapter, we will focus on a new way of thinking about medicine—percutaneous hydrotomy.

CHAPTER 3

A New Way of Thinking about Medicine—Percutaneous Hydrotomy

The history of percutaneous hydrotomy is fascinating and rooted in advancements in European medicine during the Industrial Revolution. During the 1800s, doctors were faced with treating diseases such as malnutrition, cholera, kwashiorkor, malaria, and tuberculosis—most of which were incurable. It was within this context that various medical techniques emerged, serving as the foundation for regenerative injection techniques like percutaneous hydrotomy.

Percutaneous hydrotomy stems from techniques utilizing mesotherapy, oligotherapy, tumescent anesthesia, hypodermoclysis, and regenerative medicine.

- Mesotherapy, which originated in France and derives from the Greek term *mesos* (middle), uses microinjections of

pharmaceuticals, vitamins, and other preparations into the skin and subcutaneous tissues. Mesotherapy only became possible with the invention of injectable needles.
- Oligotherapy involves treating diseases with bioavailable forms of trace minerals. In the late 1800s, trace minerals discovered by chemists were used to treat many kinds of ailments of that time.
- Tumescent anesthesia is the placement of large volumes of saline and dilute local anesthesia in the subcutaneous tissues. This technique facilitates pain management and local anesthesia during procedures.
- Hypodermoclysis is a decades-old practice involving the subcutaneous infusion of fluids into the body. It is safe, straightforward, and effective for administering fluids and delivering medications.
- Regenerative medicine, as discussed in chapter 1, involves prolotherapy, platelet-rich plasma injections (PRP), adult stem cell injections, perineural superficial injections, and saline injections.
- Together, these techniques and principles from the basis of percutaneous hydrotomy and aim to treat the causes and bring back function to those suffering with chronic pain.

The History of the Percutaneous Hydrotomy Technique

At the beginning of the twentieth century, Colonel René Quinton, a French biologist, published a book called *L'eau de Mer Milieu Organique*, which translates to "Marine Water, Organic Environment" (Quinton, 1912). His contributions sparked a scientific revolution, paving new and innovative avenues for treating patients. Quinton was a man of diverse talents—he was a physiologist, researcher, author, soldier, and aviator. Even the Wright brothers once wrote to Quinton asking for his expertise in designing airplane wings (Renard, 1925).

Quinton gained recognition for his groundbreaking approach of injecting sterilized marine water subcutaneously to treat diseases like tuberculosis, syphilis, herpes, malnutrition, kwashiorkor, typhoid fever, gastrointestinal diseases, and skin disorders (Fortan, 1925). His results were nothing short of miraculous. He called this marine water the "milieu organique." Quinton developed a method for sterilizing marine water and making it safe to administer through subcutaneous and intravenous injections to infants, children, and adults (Fortan, 1925). He saved thousands of infants worldwide with his marine serum treatments when medicine had few good answers for children dying from malnutrition, dehydration, and cholera. Generations of young patients were saved from certain death and were thus referred to as the "Babies of Quinton." Dr. Theodore Boutillier also described the marine water treatment given by subcutaneous injections in children with excellent results. He was careful to state that the Quinton serum isn't a panacea, but a valuable treatment for children with marasmus, cholera, and malnutrition (Boutillier, 1910). By 1910 about seventy clinics had opened in France, dedicated to dispensing Quinton's marine treatments. These clinical results were published and the subjects followed for over fifteen years (Jarricot, 1921). Thousands of photos and testimonies exist from doctors who administered this marine serum, which was later called "the plasma of Quinton."

René Quinton graduated from college at age fifteen with a bachelor of science degree, became a biologist, and started working as a research assistant and performing research at the College of France in Paris; this laid the foundation for his groundbreaking

A New Way of Thinking about Medicine

discoveries in the field of marine water. His studies revealed that marine water contains many of the same constituents as blood and other body tissues (Quinton, 1912). This led him to hypothesize that life indeed originated from the ocean, a concept that resonates with the beliefs of many contemporary scientists (NASA Laboratory, 2014). Quinton believed that the "milieu vital" was the extracellular fluid bathing the cells and providing nourishment. He called it the "milieu interior"—the blood and plasma. He documented seventy-eight different minerals in marine water, similar to human serum; he performed hundreds of experiments in his laboratory, injecting animals with sterilized marine water. In one of his most famous experiments, he removed a significant amount of blood from dogs and injected them with the same volume of isotonic marine water. Astonishingly, all the dogs did well throughout the experiment, were not agitated, and had no gastrointestinal or urinary issues; they were described as trotting about the following day, living many years after the experiments (Quinton, 1912). Quinton described procuring marine water from ten to thirty meters below the surface at a specific time of day. The marine water was then transported to Paris in glass containers without being sterilized. The marine water was then cold-filtered and mixed with distilled water to make it isotonic, or similar to human plasma.

Quinton's insights and pioneering work challenged conventional notions of the body's internal environment, and he highlighted the parallels between marine water and human physiology. René Quinton's remarkable journey was cut short when he died unexpectedly of an apparent heart attack on July 11, 1925, at only fifty-eight years of age. Every newspaper in France wrote about his death, which prompted one of the largest funeral processions in the history of France (Fortan, 1925). The French prime minister delivered the eulogy for a man most of us have never heard of; a man whose lifework saved untold numbers of lives. Thousands of mothers and the children he saved were standing in the streets of Paris during his cortège. French presidents, generals, physicians, surgeons, engineers, and colleagues wrote about him after his death. One doctor wrote, "I remember the testimony of the parents of thousands of children who were treated and saved by this marine serum created by Quinton, and thanks to him, many avoided getting sick and even dying" (Fortan, 1925).

Despite the medical establishment being skeptical of René Quinton's discoveries, he persisted. Science and war exist in similar environments. Science is truly the war of humanity. Biologists must discover the invisible and possess the same virtues, heroism, and intelligence to overcome enemies. The laboratory is the battlefield that requires the same courage, and the microscope is akin to the cannons used to advance in position. Quinton exemplified all these qualities, saving thousands, serving his country, and creating stimulating debate. He was held in the same esteem as Lavoisier (the father of chemistry), Claude Bernard (the father of physiology), and Louis Pasteur (the father of microbiology). The works of Quinton are among the elite.

The Evolution of Therapeutic Injections to Relieve Pain

The history of therapeutic injections into the skin date back to ancient Chinese, Roman, and Indian medicine. Hippocrates (400 BC) used a local cactus application for shoulder pain (Sivagnanam, 2010). Over two thousand years ago, Chinese acupuncturists healed patients. The practice of injections is clearly documented in the 1650s. Sir Christopher Wren used a syringe made of an animal bladder fixed to a goose quill to inject wine and opium into the veins of dogs (Norn, 2006).

A New Way of Thinking about Medicine

Following the invention of the hollow needle in the nineteenth century, the injection of substances became commonplace. In 1847, Karl Baunscheidt hypothesized that a drug could act on the body if superficially injected into the dermis at a depth of two millimeters (Sivagnanam, 2010). In 1853, Scottish physician Alexander Wood injected the first dose of intradermal morphine to induce relief for many painful conditions. In 1860, Bartolomeo Guala began practicing systematic hypodermic (below the dermis) injections in a hospital. Subcutaneous infusion was first described in 1865 for treating dehydration in patients with cholera. This procedure involved fluids being injected into the subcutaneous tissues, which were then absorbed into the circulation (Day, 1913). In 1867, Nepalese physician Gaetano Primavera conducted experiments to assess drug absorption in the urine after hypodermic administration (Mammucari, 2020). That same year, the London Medical Society, published an article about hypodermic injections highlighting the advantages including the increases safety and speed of administration, the production of a physiological effect with a lower dose compared to other methods, the certainty of the effects, the ease of application, and the absence of certain side-effects seen with other drugs. The fields of pain medicine, intravenous therapy, and vaccines were all born out of the invention of hypodermic needles.

That same year, the London Medical Society, citing hypodermic injections, wrote, 'The speed, intensity, and safety of the action, the production of an effect with a lower dose compared to other administration methods, the certainty of the effects, the ease of application, and the absence of certain disagreeable side effects of other drugs.' The fields of pain medicine, intravenous therapy, and vaccines all emerged from the invention of hypodermic needles.

Stopping Pain

In 1870, doctors injected distilled water into the dermis of soldiers during the Franco-Prussian War to relieve arthritic pain. Ophthalmologist Karl Koller initially reported the use of cocaine for local pain management in 1884 (Rotunda, 2006). Alfred Einhorn discovered a novel anesthetic called procaine, or novocaine, or new cocaine. Albert Lemaire, a Belgian physician, relieved trigeminal neuralgia, a nerve disease causing extreme face pain, using local procaine injections. French surgeon René Leriche injected procaine into inflamed tendons and the stellate ganglia, which is a cluster of nerves affecting pain in the face, head, and arms. William Halsted, an American surgeon, reported in 1885 that sterile water caused local anesthesia (Imber, 2010). In 1894, Pietro Orlandini, a Venetian doctor, used dermal punctures to treat some forms of localized pain. Prolotherapy began in the 1930s. Dr. George Hackett started using saline and dextrose as a healing agent for damaged tendons and ligaments (Shipley, 2013). In 1941, George D. Gammon and Isaac Starr published the analgesic effect of sterile water injection into the skin over or near the pain (Mammucari, 2020). Platelet-rich plasma (PRP) has been used since the 1950s to help heal bone grafts. In 1958, Michel Pistor proposed the term "mesotherapy" (Pistor, 1998). In 2004, Sergio Maggiori, analyzing preclinical and clinical trials, proposed the term "local intradermal therapy" (LIT) to emphasize that superficial inoculation allowed the clinical effect with a lower dose of a drug (Mammucari, 2020).

Karl Braunscheidt	First drug dermal injection (2 millimeters)	1847
Alexander Wood	First injection of dermic morphine	1853
Bartolomeo Primavera	Systematic hypodermic treatment in a hospital	1860

A New Way of Thinking about Medicine

Gaetano Primavera	First experiment to assess the degree of drug absorption in the urine after hypodermic administration	1867
London Medical Society	Definition of "hypodermic injections"	1867
Physicians during the Franco-Prussian war	Doctors injected distilled water into the dermis for pain	1870
William Halstead	Intradermal inoculation of sterile water induces local anesthesia	1885
Pietro Orlandini	Dermal punctures for pain	1894
George Gammon and Isaac Starr	Analgesic effect of sterile water inoculation into the skin for pain	1941
Michel Pistor	Proposed the term "mesotherapy"	1958
Bernard Guez	Proposed the term "percutaneous hydrotomy"	1990
Sergio Maggiori	Proposed the term "local intradermal therapy" (LIT)	2004

Table 1. A timeline of the invention of dermal injections, mesotherapy, and percutaneous hydrotomy.

The Creation of Percutaneous Hydrotomy

Percutaneous hydrotomy was created from the combination of the following disciplines. All disciplines have numerous studies showing their safety and efficacy.

- Mesotherapy—the administration of small quantities of drugs in a localized area
- Oligotherapy—the action of trace minerals at the cellular level

- Tumescent anesthesia technique—the safe use of local anesthetics diluted in large quantities of physiological saline
- Hypodermoclysis—the subcutaneous injection of fluids given safely in terms of hydration and for the slow and dilute absorption of drugs
- Water—for its ability to diffuse and as a vehicle to deliver vitamins, minerals, and medications

Mesotherapy

Mesotherapy is the infiltration of the superficial layer of skin for preventive, curative, and rehabilitative purposes (Mammucari, 2020). The word derives from Greek *mesos* [middle] and *therapeia* [therapy] and means a minimally invasive technique of subcutaneous delivery of pharmaceuticals, homeopathic preparations, plant extracts, and vitamins. Local action is the first lesson, and the skin acts as a natural time-release system.

Dr. Michel Pistor (1924–2003) was a genius on the edge of medicine (Sivagnanum, 2010). Dr. Pistor envisioned that treating the target problem at the anatomical site would lower the required dose of medications and their adverse side effects. The history of how mesotherapy came into practice is fascinating. After finishing general medicine studies at the Faculty of Medicine in Paris, Pistor began practicing in a small country village near Paris called Bray-et-Lû. It all began when he administered the local anesthetic procaine to a patient to halt an acute asthma attack. While it did little for the asthma attack, it improved the patient's profound hearing loss (Pistor, 1976). Soon after, Pistor began experimenting with subcutaneous injections of procaine around the ears of patients with hearing loss and discovered that many could hear the village church bells again. Scores of patients came to Pistor; many people showed

A New Way of Thinking about Medicine

improvements, while others did not. Also, many reported improvements in eczema, tinnitus, and TMJ pain. Dr. Pistor then began injecting around the lesion area in question. Later, this was recognized as the original application of mesotherapy (Pistor, 1979).

In 1953, Dr. Mario Lebel engineered a 3 mm needle that facilitated the subcutaneous delivery of medications. Pistor and Lebel experimented with different medications for several indications. Pistor then coined the term "mesotherapy," focusing on local drug delivery rather than on oral medications (Pistor, 1976).

In 1964, Pistor founded the French Society of Mesotherapy. He published "Therapeutic Challenge," introducing the notion of local injection of drugs: "little, rarely and in the right place," setting the foundations for mesotherapy. In 1987, the French National Academy of Medicine acknowledged mesotherapy as an official medical specialty.

Mesotherapy has gained widespread success in France and other regions worldwide, especially for cosmetic applications. In 2005, the French social security system established a standardized classification of medical procedures describing mesotherapy for pain relief (Bonnet, 2012; D'Alloz-Bourguignon, 1980). Michel Pistor died in 2003 and was posthumously awarded France's highest distinction, the Legion of Honor. Practiced worldwide, mesotherapy is quite popular throughout Europe and South America. In the United States, it isn't taught in medical schools, and there are no federal or state regulations defining its scope of practice. Many healthcare providers, including physicians and non-physicians, learn mesotherapy through hands-on training courses, often in Europe (Bonnet, 2012). Although the US Food and Drug Administration (FDA) hasn't approved mesotherapy as a procedure, many of the medications used in mesotherapy are FDA approved; common examples are Botox and soft tissue filler injections.

Stopping Pain

Dr. Guez pioneered the development of percutaneous hydrotomy through local injections of physiologic saline, local anesthetics, NSAIDs, vasodilators, minerals, and vitamins into painful areas. He developed his ideas to treat chronic back pain utilizing mesotherapy techniques by injecting saline and medications into the subcutaneous tissues of the back, initially naming the procedure "mesotherapy and hydration." Depending on the specific chronic disease, he found that administering 10, 20, and even 500 milliliters was effective, safe, and well tolerated. After fifteen years of observation and refinement, Dr. Guez would coin the term "percutaneous hydrotomy."

When Dr. Guez talks about his training with Dr. Pistor, it's like a good history lesson, and everyone listens. Drs. Pistor and Guez communicated often about mesotherapy and hydration to treat chronic pain. In his writings about the future of mesotherapy into the third millennium, Dr. Pistor referred to the technique as "surface mesotherapy" (Guez, 2021). They often discussed research ideas, such as the potential of water to heal and cure diseases. For example, they hypothesized about using percutaneous hydrotomy to shrink tumors using hypertonic saline. With a radio-guided needle, it would be possible to place the tip near the tumor and inject hypertonic saline in hopes of locally destroying it. Drs. Guez and Pistor were certainly ahead of their time.

A crucial point to emphasize is that percutaneous hydrotomy is a technique based on mesotherapy principles and hydration, and it relies on the utilization of mesotherapy techniques to attain its desired outcomes. While it is a new discipline, it is a continuation of the groundbreaking work done—and proven effective time and time again—by Dr. Pistor. In 2006, Dr. Guez formed the International Society of Percutaneous Hydrotomy and developed training courses to educate fellow healthcare practitioners. (Guez, 2020).

A New Way of Thinking about Medicine

Mesotherapy and Fat Loss

Mesotherapy received its initial advance into the American consciousness when the American singer Roberta Flack attributed her remarkable transformation to mesotherapy (combined with a comprehensive diet and exercise routine) (Matarasso, 2009). She was given injections of deoxycholate (a natural detergent) and phosphatidylcholine (a natural phospholipid), which are designed to dissolve subcutaneous fat.

Michel Pistor performed clinical research and founded the field of mesotherapy for medical rather than aesthetic purposes. It's essential to distinguish mesotherapy from phosphatidylcholine injections. Several lay and peer-reviewed publications have reported that subcutaneous phosphatidylcholine injections are efficacious in treating localized collections of fat (Rotunda, 2007). However, the colloquial definition of mesotherapy (seen commonly in advertisements) describes a method to reduce cellulite, treat fat, or refresh the aging face. Wellness centers and medical spas have embraced mesotherapy as a novel treatment for cellulite, fat loss, and photoaging (sun damage). The French Society of Mesotherapy and Percutaneous Hydrotomy recognizes its use as a treatment for various conditions but doesn't mention its use in plastic surgery (Matarasso, 2009; Rotunda, 2007).

Oligotherapy

Oligotherapy is a biochemical approach that addresses trace mineral deficiencies and helps us understand the cellular basis of disease—the biological terrain. *Oligos*, in Greek, means a very tiny quantity.

Stopping Pain

In the early 1900s, French chemist Gabriel Bertrand, who first characterized laccase in 1894, noted that certain biological materials associated with laccase activity contained significant manganese, a trace element he studied as a cofactor in enzymatic processes (Picard, 1983).

At the Institut Pasteur, he showed that a lack of dietary manganese interrupted growth, a hotly debated finding at that time. Bertrand's research was immediately applied to undiagnosable disease conditions, which were recognized to be because of a lack of certain trace minerals. He identified these trace element enzyme cofactors and called them "oligo" elements. In 1919, French physician Dr. Jean Sutter treated tuberculosis using an ionized solution of copper and manganese and found that it accelerated wound healing (Nielson, 1990). Later, in the 1930s, French physician Jacques Menetrier demonstrated that oligo elements could effectively treat biochemical dysfunctions, basing his findings on over 75,000 patient cases. In the 1970s, Dr. Henry Picard developed mesotherapy techniques for injecting trace minerals to treat hip osteoarthritis and performed clinical trials on over 50,000 patients; his results were positive in about 85 percent of his cases. He published numerous articles and a book called *Vaincre l'Arthrose*, which translates to *Beating Arthritis* (Picard, 1983).

Oligotherapy involves the use of tiny doses of natural forms of trace minerals that are a powerful modality for treating many conditions, including chronic diseases, infections, cardiovascular disease, circulatory disorders, and neurological conditions (Nielsen, 1990). The deficiency of these minerals causes the appearance of diseases such as osteoarthritis.

Oligotherapy is a therapeutic approach providing the body with minerals that are indispensable for cellular enzymatic

A New Way of Thinking about Medicine

functions. This functional therapeutic modality requires using highly bioavailable trace elements in precisely measured small doses. Carbon, hydrogen, oxygen, and nitrogen, along with bioavailable oligo elements, work in the body by normalizing enzyme and hormonal functions and regulating homeostasis. This approach maintains optimal health and makes it possible to act on the root causes of disease.

Specific trace element deficiencies become apparent only when the body is stressed, increasing the need for those elements. Recent findings have supported this with selenium (Nutrition & Health, 1996). Like selenium, the trace elements boron and copper are of nutritional significance. Research shows that boron and calcium are involved in bone metabolism (Rondanelli, 2020). Copper deficiency in humans varies with amino acid and carbohydrate composition in the diet (Nielson, 1990). Chromium, molybdenum, nickel, arsenic, and vanadium may be of nutritional significance, especially under stressful conditions. For example, many patients with psoriatic and rheumatoid arthritis are prescribed methotrexate, a medication used to manage the pain and inflammation. Methotrexate alters the blood levels of zinc and copper in humans (Gao, 2021).

The ionized trace elements include bismuth, cobalt, fluoride, copper chromium, iodine, lithium, magnesium, manganese, molybdenum, phosphorus, potassium, selenium, sulfur, and zinc. Oligo elements, or trace elements, derive from metals, except for calcium, fluoride, magnesium, phosphorus, potassium, selenium, and sulfur. Percutaneous hydrotomy is well placed to deliver oligo elements to facilitate cellular regeneration from disease states and damaged tissues (Guez, 2020).

Tumescent Local Anesthesia

The term tumescence, by definition, is the state of being swollen, and anesthesia is the use of medicines to prevent pain (analgesia). The idea of aesthetic medicine was advanced in the 1990s by doctors Pierre François Fournier (France) and Jeffrey Klein (the United States) when they developed tumescent anesthesia, which involves injecting local anesthetic and physiological saline subcutaneously to produce anesthesia for liposuction and other aesthetic procedures (Fournier, 1989). Tumescent anesthesia includes various amounts of saline, dilute local anesthetics, analgesics, and vasoconstrictive agents.

The idea of injecting large volumes of dilute anesthetic solutions into the subcutaneous tissue was known as "massive infiltration" (Welch, 1998). Various solutions, propulsion devices, flexible needles, multiple formulas, and many applications of the technique were described and illustrated in several standard American surgical textbooks from the early 1900s (Hanke, 2021). A Russian surgeon named Aleksandr Vishnevsky developed a technique in the 1930s called "Local Anesthesia by Creeping Infiltration Method," aiming to create a large, anesthetized, bloodless field using only regionally injected solutions to avoid general anesthesia. Italian physician Fischer published the first written description of liposuction in 1977 (Hanke, 2021). A few years later, the French surgeons Yves-Gerard Illouz and Fournier popularized liposuction using blunt-tipped cannulas (Hartung, 2023). Since that time, the solutions used for infiltrating tissue have developed considerably. In fact, from the late 1970s onward, it's difficult to document all the significant changes and improvements in tumescent anesthesia (Hanke, 2021).

In 1977, Illouz advanced the tumescent technique, which involved injecting small amounts of saline, lidocaine, hyaluronidase, and epinephrine into the subcutaneous fat (Hartung, 2023). The current technique of tumescent anesthesia, popularized by the American physician Jeffrey Klein, has grown from the developments of local anesthetic agents and various infusion devices over the last 110 years. Dr. Klein was persistent in his belief that liposuction could be done safely without a general anesthetic. Tumescent anesthesia increased patient safety and decreased the high costs of operating rooms (Klein, 1993). In our current era, ~~Hamacher and~~ Dr. Jeffrey Klein deserves credit for reintroducing this technique and establishing parameters for lidocaine toxicity.

Hypodermoclysis

Hypodermoclysis is a technique used to safely infuse large quantities of physiological solutions and drugs into the subcutaneous tissues through a needle. It's a safe, effective, acceptable, and efficient treatment modality for mild to moderate dehydration in the geriatric and pediatric populations (JAMA 1952, Dardaine, 2005; Steiner, 1998; Berger, 1984; Farrand, 1996; Remington, 2007; Adem, 2021). Also called "interstitial infusion," it is the subcutaneous administration of saline and glucose solutions; it could also be called "mesotherapy and hydration," as Dr. Guez originally described it. Many medical societies, including the International Society of Percutaneous Hydrotomy, and healthcare providers support using subcutaneous infusions (Spandorfer, 2011).

The earliest mention of hypodermoclysis dates back to 1865, when Italian physician Arnaldo Catani treated dehydration in patients with cholera (Giordano, 2018; *Lancet*, 1885). Certainly, René Quinton is among the practitioners who used subcutaneous infusions to save patients from dehydration. Dr. J. R. Day published a report in 1913 on subcutaneous rehydration to treat infantile diarrhea (Miller, 1913; Day, 1913). In fact, Burford reported that Day had actually used Quinton's marine serum in many of his patients (Burford, 1913).

Hypodermoclysis enjoyed widespread use throughout the 1940s and 1950s. Subcutaneous rehydration therapy, originally referred to as hypodermoclysis, shows promise as an alternative to intravenous fluid administration for treating dehydration (Giordano, 2018). The chief advantages of hypodermoclysis over intravenous infusion are that it's safe, inexpensive, easy to perform, and can be administered by nonmedical personnel with minimal supervision in the home or in the office. The Infusion Therapy Standards of Practice recommends considering subcutaneous access for the administration of isotonic solutions and other infusion therapies (AAP, 1996). Ideal medications for subcutaneous administration are those that are hydrosoluble and have neutral pH, low viscosity, and low molecular weight such as baclofen, buprenorphine, hydromorphone, ketorolac, ketamine, methadone, morphine, and tramadol (Bruno, 2015). Irritating additives, such as propylene glycol, glycerin, and ethanol, should be avoided, as these can be associated with adverse reactions and discomfort. The enzyme hyaluronidase can be added to improve fluid absorption (AAP, 1996).

Percutaneous Hydrotomy

The practice of percutaneous hydrotomy is, first, an area of general medicine that attempts to rethink the approach to pain and disease. No longer is it sufficient to base a treatment solely on allopathic principles; a consideration of the biological terrain (discussed in chapter 5) is essential for the desired outcome. Percutaneous hydrotomy consists of injecting a physiologic saline solution into the

A New Way of Thinking about Medicine

intradermal or subcutaneous spaces. The term derives from ancient Greek ὕδριος (*hudrios*), meaning water, and the verb τέμνειν (*temnein*), meaning to cut or to incise—in other words, pushing and infiltrating water into organs and tissues. Despite the diversity of these practices, few people have taken an interest in the impact of water on our bodies.

The injection of the hydrotomy solution results in temporary swelling of the soft tissues creating a tumescent state or "hydrotomy cushion." The hydrotomy cushion is synonymous with mesotherapy and hydration, or the tumescent technique in aesthetic medicine, or hypodermoclysis in geriatric medicine. It's recognizable by temporary skin swelling at the local level. Slow local diffusion makes it possible to treat a lesion in a targeted manner. Percutaneous hydrotomy allows local treatment using low doses of diluted drugs and with minimal side effects. The action is precise and focuses on the functional causes of the disease.

Percutaneous hydrotomy is a regenerative medicine technique, meaning that it operates at the cellular level. This process involves water, electrolytes, trace elements, minerals, magnesium, vitamins, organic silica, amino acids, and certain medications with the goal of rebalancing the cellular constituents so that the body can find a healthy equilibrium. This concept of regenerative medicine has been the subject of many studies in aesthetic medicine. Using the most abundant chemical element in our body—water—it intervenes at different physiological, biological, and biochemical levels. Water has a neuroanatomical action, meaning it acts on the nerves and generates mechanical plasticity; water is the best conductor of an electric current. Numerous studies have shown that water possesses therapeutic properties and is not merely a placebo (Altman 2016; Zhang, 2008; Scott, 2019).

Stopping Pain

> ### Clinical Case: Madame F., fifty-nine years old
> #### Shoulder Pain
>
> Since June 2018, I have suffered from adhesive capsulitis in my left shoulder, unable to lift my arm vertically or behind my back, followed by intense pain, especially at night. In November, my physiotherapist aggravated my shoulder and referred me to an osteopathic physician, which didn't help. In December, a rheumatologist performed a cortisone infiltration, which temporarily calmed the pain (three weeks). In February 2019, a second physiotherapist specializing in shoulder pathologies brought some improvement, but the stiffness and pain remained.
>
> Finally, I was referred to a clinic which offered me percutaneous hydrotomy. In March 2019, I had my first percutaneous injection hydrotomy session. I noticed a significant improvement, and my arm and my shoulder felt noticeably lighter. Two days later, the pain was gone. To date, I have had four percutaneous hydrotomy sessions, which have resulted in marked improvement in my stiffness and pain and a positive evolution of my range of motion (approved and observed by the physiotherapist). The pains have also disappeared at night, and my days pass with a feeling of renewal.

Cellular Energy

On an energetic and fundamental level, percutaneous hydrotomy recharges the cellular energy metabolism via the Krebs cycle. Water recharges the connective tissue (collagen) and facilitates regeneration and detoxification which will facilitate exchange with other cells. Dr. Guez called this process a "washout" or "therapeutic lavage."

A New Way of Thinking about Medicine

Water is the best vehicle for delivering therapeutics at the cellular level. This process promotes hydration and diluting of local chemical mediators of tissue inflammation, which manifests as swelling, edema, pain, redness, and warmth. Water is an anti-inflammatory without side effects. To put it simply, water extinguishes fire.

Skin

The skin plays a vital role in the percutaneous hydrotomy technique. It's the primary filtration organ and creates a therapeutic reservoir where large amounts of fluids can be placed. It facilitates the passage of injected products while protecting the deep organs (liver, kidney, brain, heart), which are usually affected by conventional treatments. Two advantages of the subcutaneous route are (1) lower doses of medications, and (2) the treatment can be directed at the level of the lesion, making the therapeutic effect much more effective. Unlike traditional mesotherapy, the injected products are diluted to avoid side effects. Koulakis and colleagues showed that tumescent injections disperse fluids volumetrically and maintain elevated local concentrations of additives for several hours (Koulakis, 2020). In the tumescent state, tissue permeability dramatically increases, enhancing fluid and medication dispersal. Percutaneous hydrotomy gives the cells the micronutrition needed for regeneration so that the organs can repair themselves and rebalance homeostasis.

The next chapter will focus on the fundamental units of percutaneous hydrotomy. An understanding of these concepts is crucial to the mechanisms of how percutaneous hydrotomy heals chronic diseases.

Part Two
The Science

CHAPTER 4

The Five Foundations of Percutaneous Hydrotomy

Conventional medicine views people in terms of their disease—a one-size-fits-all model. It focuses on naming a disease, seeing a specialist, and prescribing a pill for that disease rather than trying to prevent it in the first place. For example, a patient with neck pain will see a spine specialist, obtain X-rays, be prescribed pain and anti-inflammatory medications, and schedule a follow-up appointment.

Percutaneous hydrotomy thinks differently. Rather than focusing only on the symptoms and the names of diseases, we consider what's causing the dysfunction, and then how we can reestablish proper function of the cells, nerves, circulatory system, immune system, and cellular energy. We accomplish this by thinking of chronic disease in units of competency, which all have specific roles in the equilibrium of the organism.

A unit of competency can be defined as a segment of a treatment or skill set that a medical practitioner is expected to master. Units are building blocks in the construction of one's professional capacity to perform a task such as percutaneous hydrotomy effectively and safely. There may be a range where these units of competence are applied to different contexts or conditions, such as knee pain or neuropathic pain. For example, chronic neuropathic pain involves all five units of competency.

The Five Units of Competency

The five units of competency have a specific role in the balance and the equilibrium of the human body.

1. Fundamental Unit: the cells and the biological terrain
2. Circulatory Unit: the blood vessels
3. Neurological Unit: the nerves
4. Immune Unit: the natural defenses
5. Energy Unit: cellular energy

In the context of percutaneous hydrotomy, we have found it simpler to explain the physiological concepts of percutaneous hydrotomy in competency units. The Merriam-Webster dictionary defines competency as the quality of having sufficient knowledge, judgment, skill, or strength for a particular duty. A competency unit, as it pertains to the practice of percutaneous hydrotomy, defines the organism's structure, energy, and function and emphasizes the need for a wide range of knowledge of the pathology and the treatment options. For example, the largest organ is the skin, and it's a common denominator of the fundamental, circulatory, neurological, immune, and energy units.

Various physicians developed the key competency units.

The Five Foundations of Percutaneous Hydrotomy

- Dr. Yannick Huteau developed the fundamental competency unit (Pistor, 1979).
- Dr. Andre Dalloz-Bourguignon developed the first ideas for the circulatory, neurological, and immune competencies (Dalloz-Bourguignon, 1990).
- Dr. Jean-Pierre Multedo further developed the concepts of the circulatory unit, which he called the third circulation (Multedo, 2018).
- The fifth unit of competency, the energy unit, was developed in the 1980s by Dr. Daniel Ballesteros. He based his theories on spectrophotometric images after injecting trace minerals and other oligo elements.

Percutaneous hydrotomy acts on one or more of these five competency units to restore physiological balance and energy. Their dysfunctions will promote the appearance of a group of diseases and their symptoms. Percutaneous hydrotomy uses the five competencies to serve as a base for the indication and treatment of the diseases in question.

The Fundamental Unit

The word *fundamental* defines the cells and their environment, which includes the biological terrain, water, the cellular matrix, proteins, DNA, and collagen. Your body constantly sends electrical impulses, pumping blood, filtering urine, digesting food, making proteins, and storing fat—all things we never even think about. You can do all this because of the fundamental unit—cells. Cells are specialized factories full of machinery designed to accomplish the business of life. Every living thing, from whales to archaebacteria inside volcanoes, is made of cells.

Stopping Pain

Cells come in all shapes and sizes. Nerve cells in giant squids can reach up to 12 meters (39 feet) in length, while human eggs (the largest human cells) are about 0.1 mm in diameter. Fungal cell walls are made from the same stuff as lobster shells. However, despite this vast range in size, shape, and function, all these little factories have similar machinery. Think about what a factory needs to effectively function: a building, a product, and the means to make that product. All cells have membranes (the building), DNA (the various blueprints), and ribosomes (the production line), so they can make proteins (the product).

An organelle (a cell's internal organ) is a membrane-bound structure found within a cell. You can think of organelles as smaller rooms within the factory, with specialized conditions to help these rooms carry out their tasks. The cytoplasm, structured water within the cell membrane, houses the organelles and is the location of most of the action in cells.

Water constitutes the interior and the exterior of the cell environment. Healthy cells tightly regulate water; diseased cells do not (Marques, 2022; Morishita, 2019). Water dysregulation results in cell dysfunction, less energy production, and even cell death. Consequently, many diseases, including arthritis, fibrosis, sclerosis, and necrosis, are degenerative in nature. Dehydration is an example of water dysregulation and leads to the appearance of degenerative diseases, such as arthritis, degeneration, and aging; this is why painful arthritic knees are often swollen.

Even during sleep, your body is working to maintain balance. This is called homeostasis, which means the body maintains internal stability to compensate for environmental changes. Cell regulation involves constant formation and destruction, a process known as apoptosis, that is a normal part of aging. When cells stop dividing and

The Five Foundations of Percutaneous Hydrotomy

don't undergo apoptosis, these are called senescent cells. These damaged cells resist the body's usual system of disposal and then linger; they remain and continue to release inflammatory chemicals that can damage other cells and even turn cancerous. Restoring a healthy cellular environment allows the senescent cells to move toward apoptosis.

Aging is a complex reality involving both genetic and environmental processes. Despite numerous theories, no one has ever discovered why we age (Jin, 2010). For example, with age we progressively lose muscle mass, which results in a loss of function. This occurs in part because the intracellular level of amino acids decreases, specifically glutamine. Amino acid transport to the muscle cells is a major determinant in muscle and protein regulation (Timmerman, 2008). Amino acids (arginine, leucine, valine, isoleucine, alanine, and glutamine) support cellular regeneration and DNA synthesis.

The goals of percutaneous hydrotomy are to address the cells and their environment by exposing the lesion or area of pain to physiologic water, which becomes the vehicle for trace minerals, vitamins, anti-inflammatories, and amino acids. The treatment of this fundamental unit in percutaneous hydrotomy includes hydration with physiological saline solutions and cellular micronutrition containing:

- Injectable trace elements (oligotherapy) in small quantities (zinc, copper, manganese, cobalt, iodine, and selenium) for their biocatalytic action, which replenishes minerals, according to the work of Dr. Picard (Picard, 1983)
- Injectable vitamins: Vitamin A (cell regeneration), B-complex vitamins (cell metabolism), vitamins C and E (antioxidants and anti-free radicals), vitamin D (skin regeneration), and vitamin K (circulatory system and bones)

Stopping Pain

- Organic silica: Attracts water and supports cellular plasticity
- Amino acids: The experience of using amino acids in percutaneous hydrotomy has been positive. We have observed considerable progress in degenerative diseases, such as osteoarthritis. Amino acids are important for deoxyribonucleic acid (DNA) homeostasis, and with age, the quantity and quality of these amino acids decrease, coupled with dehydration, resulting in suboptimal cellular function. DNA serves as the photocopier of cellular information—the risk of genetic mutations (coding errors) increases with age and sometimes becomes the source of cancer or disease. Delivering water and amino acids to the cells reinforces genetic coding and protein synthesis.
- Magnesium: An essential aspect of cellular health and energy, participating in hundreds of enzymatic reactions. It also improves the transmission of nerve impulses and decreases nerve irritation.
- EDTA (for medical use): Chelating agents, such as EDTA, are an important aspect of percutaneous hydrotomy. EDTA binds or chelates heavy metals such as lead, mercury, and calcium, allowing them to be excreted in the urine; it's also effective in mobilizing the diseased calcium formations, such as in osteophytes.

Chronic disease results from changes in cell function, energy, replication, and micronutrition which result in the development of degenerative diseases such as arthritis, fibrosis, and cell death. Percutaneous hydrotomy utilizes different interventions to target these underlying issues. Using physiologic water, for example, promotes cellular hydration and improves function. Oligotherapy, which involves the

The Five Foundations of Percutaneous Hydrotomy

use of bioavailable forms of trace minerals, supports cellular processes. Local anesthetics can provide analgesia, helping to break the cycle of chronic pain. Chelating agents can be used to remove heavy metals and mobilize diseased calcium deposits.

> ### Clinical Case: Mr. B., eighty years old
> #### Back Pain
>
> I'm a former marathon runner and I have a narrow lumbar canal and multiple herniated discs (four levels), likely from my years of running. I was scheduled for a lumbar spine operation, but following a heart attack, I underwent open-heart surgery in 2017. Thus, the back operation was postponed. Following my heart operation, I walked more but with difficulty, frequently stopping to relieve my back pain. According to my neurosurgeon, without an operation within six months, paralysis of my legs would be the result. Having learned that there was a solution called percutaneous hydrotomy, I decided to take a risk and am happy to report that I'm walking better and better after about a year. I receive percutaneous hydrotomy treatments once a month. Thanks to this great treatment, I'm living life again and I won't have to resort to an operation in the long term.

The Circulatory Unit

The circulatory unit encompasses the 60,000 miles of arteries, veins, capillaries, arterials, venules, and lymphatics that supply the body with oxygen, nutrients, water, and much more. Dysfunction within the microcirculatory system results in diseases like heart attacks, erectile dysfunction, nonhealing chronic wounds, venous stasis ulcers, pressure ulcers, and diabetic wounds. With chronic disease, the small arteries may gradually obstruct and decrease pressure, causing a lack of oxygen and nutrient delivery. We refer to these as areas of cell death as micro-infarctions. A common example of infarction is a heart attack, which results in dead cardiac muscle cells. Heart attacks result from blocked coronary arteries, mainly from inflammation, poor diet, smoking, and lack of exercise (Henein, 2022).

Dysfunction of the circulatory unit may cause diseases to appear where blood circulation is no longer adequate, usually at the level of the small vessels—memory problems, migraines, tinnitus, balance disorders, hearing loss, osteoporosis, and micro-infarction result.

Treatment of the circulatory unit in percutaneous hydrotomy includes:

- Local anesthetics
- Small doses of vasodilators, which dilate blood vessels and increase oxygenation
- Low doses of anti-inflammatories, which provide a blood-thinning antiplatelet effect or aspirin-like effect
- Melilot, a veno-lymphatic tonic used in venous insufficiency (with water retention and fat leg) or cellulitis (used mainly in Europe)

The Neurological Unit

The neurological unit includes the brain, spinal cord, and autonomic nervous system, which are the body's major controlling, regulatory, and communicating systems. This unit is the center of

The Five Foundations of Percutaneous Hydrotomy

all mental activity, including movement, thought, learning, and memory. When the cells are compromised, it affects nervous system functions:

- Intelligence, learning, emotions, and memory
- Control of the body's internal environment to maintain homeostasis (temperature regulation, heart rate, breathing)
- Voluntary control of movement
- Spinal cord functions (balance, pain, reflexes)

The reasons for these damaged cells are numerous.

- Mechanical damage—pathologic calcium called osteophytes compress the nerves exiting the spinal cord, limiting the delivery of oxygen, nutrients, and blood flow, and ultimately causing cell death. Herniated discs are another such example. The resulting symptoms are pain, tingling, electric shocks, migraines, falls, and the loss of strength.
- Metabolic (diabetes), drug (chemotherapy), viral (shingles), heavy metal toxicity (aluminum and mercury), or pesticidal (glyphosate) damage

Dysfunction of the neurological unit causes migraines, cervicalbrachial neuralgia, sciatica, carpal tunnel syndrome, and many other pathologies. Treatment protocols from a percutaneous hydrotomy perspective are aimed at the nerves, hormones, and neurotransmitters.

Superficial injections with a mesotherapy needle target the sensory nerves that exist within our skin as glial cells and the nerves in the subcutaneous tissues. These are our pain sensing nerves, which can be ultimately traced back to our spinal cord; all nerves are connected in this way. These nerves also supply sensation to blood vessels, other nerves, muscles, ligaments, tendons, joints, and cartilage. By injecting saline, local anesthetics, anti-inflammatories, magnesium, and vitamins, inflammation can be decreased and normal nerve function, restored. Tissue and growth factors are also stimulated, promoting healing.

The treatment of the neurological unit in percutaneous hydrotomy includes:

- Local anesthetics
- Vitamin B complexes (B1, B2, B3, B5, B6, B8, B9, B12) to strengthen the nerve structures
- Magnesium to reduce the hyperexcitability of diseased nerves and strengthens nerve impulses
- Heavy metal and calcium chelators to help detoxify and decrease mechanical nerve compression due to osteophytes (more commonly known as "bone spurs")

Percutaneous Hydrotomy and the Autonomic Nervous System (ANS)

The autonomic nervous system regulates the homeostatic functions of our internal organs, such as the heart, lungs, gastrointestinal tract, and sexual organs. The ANS is part of the peripheral nervous system, and branches into the sympathetic (fight or flight) and parasympathetic (rest and digest) nervous systems. We are usually unaware of the ANS because it functions without direct input from the brain. The intelligence of our bodies orchestrates billions of biochemical processes every second. Every cell emits and responds to electrochemical signals in an unimaginably complex and coordinated fashion, keeping our hearts pumping, lungs breathing, food digesting, eyes blinking, and immune system active—all without you even knowing. For example, we don't notice our blood vessels dilating or variations in our heart rates. The sympathetic and parasympathetic systems are vital in two situations: (1) emergencies that cause us to fight or flee (sympathetic) and (2) nonemergencies that allow us to rest and digest (parasympathetic). Unfortunately, our fight-or-flight system is needlessly activated every day; for example, when we are in traffic. We will return to the ANS at the end of this chapter.

> **The French Connection: A Mind-Heart-Body Connection Approach Using Percutaneous Hydrotomy**
>
> French healthcare providers Eve Lefrancq (cardiologist) and Florence Pittolo (clinical psychologist) started treating their patients using a mind-heart-body approach and percutaneous hydrotomy in 2018. A well-studied concept in cardiology, the mind-heart-body connection states that poor psychological health leads to detrimental habits such as stress, tobacco abuse, physical inactivity, and bad diet, resulting in inflammation and heart disease (Levine, 2019; Vaccarino, 2021). They followed several patients with end-stage cardiovascular disease, rheumatoid arthritis, arthritis, and diabetes. Dr. Lefrancq treats patients' cardiovascular problems using a multidisciplinary approach; in addition to standard cardiac treatments, she performs percutaneous hydrotomy treatments to address the patients' arthritis or other chronic pain issues. Dr. Pittolo

counsels these patients on their psychological health issues; more specifically, she teaches her patients to use postural and attitudinal techniques developed from her medical training. What they observed is fascinating. The adherence to cardiac medications rose to nearly 100 percent. There was a 90 percent reduction in pain and a decrease in global inflammation, excess medications (polypharmacy), and chest pain (angina) symptoms (Lefrancq, 2021). Patients decreased their use of corticosteroids and anti-inflammatories, and some stopped all medications. Cardiovascular health can indeed improve through behavioral, psychosocial, and biological changes.

The Immune Unit

A robust immune system protects us from pathogens and cancer cells by recognizing them and orchestrating their elimination. As such, our health is maintained thanks to a properly functioning immune system. The immune system unit includes the cellular and humoral immune systems, the different organs, and the cells. Cellular immunity operates without involving antibodies, whereas humoral immunity relies on antibodies. It's important to remember: (1) most diseases involve both arms of the immune system; (2) the immune system is part of the biological terrain that protects your body from bacteria, viruses, fungi, and toxins; and (3) dysfunction leads to inflammatory diseases in the mucous membranes or organs, ending in "itis" (rhinitis, sinusitis, bronchitis, colitis, cystitis, polyarthritis, otitis). Crohn's disease is an example of an autoimmune disease. In this unit, we will distinguish between cellular and humoral mediated immunity.

The Five Foundations of Percutaneous Hydrotomy

The inflammatory system plays a paramount role in our well-being. Besides its role in host defense against infectious agents and tumor cells, the inflammatory response is essential for tissue healing after injury. Dysregulation of this inflammatory process increases susceptibility to chronic diseases, infections, and cancer. Chronic inflammation is a painful condition linked with immunological disorders (Pahwa, 2023).

Allergies and Autoimmune Diseases

Our bodies are endlessly exposed to microbial agents and environmentally noxious substances that can trigger immune responses. Chronic allergies caused by pollen, dust, trees, etc., result from an antigen-antibody conflict (Maeda, 2019). Basically, the immune-incompetent organism doesn't know how to distinguish friends from enemies—it overreacts with an excess of histamine. We call this immune incompetence, which leads to the release of chemicals like histamine, causing symptoms like rhinitis, cough, asthma, eczema, and urticaria (itching). Healthcare providers counter this with antihistamines (e.g., Zyrtec or Claritin), which cause side effects such as drowsiness. The repeated use of these drugs can generate an inflammatory cascade, particularly hypersensitivity reactions (Shakouri, 2013). Autoimmune diseases are allergies to oneself and testify to the body's immune incompetence.

Percutaneous hydrotomy uses the mesovaccination technique, which aims to strengthen and reeducate the immune system. Mesovaccination has existed for more than forty years, mainly in Europe (Guez, 2021). Dr. Guez and many others have used mesovaccination to treat patients with chronic sinusitis and otitis (Guez, 2021). Mesovaccination uses small amounts of a vaccine—bacterial or viral—mixed with agents to boost and train the immune system.

Stopping Pain

Unlike traditional vaccination, which delivers larger doses into the muscle, mesovaccination involves tiny micro-injections into the skin's dermis to activate its immune defenses (Denis, 2007). The immune system unit treatment protocol includes multiple intradermal micro-injections of a diluted vaccine to stimulate the skin's immunity.

The skin is the main organ of immunity, our natural protective barrier acting as a recognition filter. By injecting tiny quantities of highly diluted vaccines, we can deliver information to the skin. The skin's immune system then develops active antigen-antibody complexes to defend itself. The vaccine effectively becomes information intended for the cells where the pathology occurs (sinuses, liver, intestines). The goal is to strengthen the immunity of local tissues while minimizing the risk (i.e., the tiny dose of the vaccine).

Currently, medicine doesn't yet know how to take advantage of the vast reservoir of antibodies made up by the skin. The addition of dilute microdoses of vaccines amplifies and multiplies the immune reaction with the appearance of antibodies. The mesovaccination technique consists of stimulating this immune-incompetent mucosa in a controlled and codified way to reset its functioning by stimulating its immune defenses with small quantities of nonspecific cell-mediated vaccines and regenerating it with vitamins and trace elements. Thus, during mesovaccination sessions, the mucosa can gain a new immunological competence and a state of regeneration, allowing it to reactivate its self-regulation mechanisms.

Dr. Guez has successfully treated many children with chronic sinus and ear infections using mesovaccination techniques. Based on his observations, he has found that typically three to six sessions are sufficient to significantly reduce and eliminate chronic infections. Dr. Guez uses about one-quarter of the usual dose in children and reports excellent results (Guez, 2021). During my training

The Five Foundations of Percutaneous Hydrotomy

with Dr. Guez, I had the opportunity to witness numerous children receiving mesovaccination treatments. Curious about the outcomes, I pointedly asked one of the mothers (in French) if the treatment truly worked. She replied, "Absolutely yes. These treatments have done wonders for my children. They used to have three to four ear and sinus infections per year and the doctors wanted to do surgery. Since they have started receiving these injections, the infections have disappeared, they no longer require antibiotics, and they no longer need surgery." This firsthand account from a mother underscores the positive impact mesovaccination can have for patients with recurrent infections.

Clinical Case: Woman, eighty-three years old

Bronchitis

Every year, I suffer from two to three severe bronchitis bouts, requiring large doses of antibiotics and long treatment periods. I have even been hospitalized for some of these situations. In December 2018, Dr. Guez offered to try mesovaccination for my severe bouts of bronchitis, and I underwent one treatment per week for three months. Since then, I no longer cough; this is the first winter I haven't had a bout of bronchitis, and I'm breathing much better. Dr. Guez has hundreds of cases like this.

The treatment of the immune unit from a percutaneous hydrotomy perspective includes the ears, nose, and throat (ENT), respiratory (lungs), liver (hepatic), gastrointestinal, and urogenital systems. Mesovaccination protocol is composed of:

Stopping Pain

- A topical local anesthetic
- Magnesium
- Organic silica
- B Vitamins
- Vaccines (small doses and highly diluted)

Achieving Vaccination with Smaller Doses of Vaccines

As Dr. Louis Pasteur once said, "the microbe is nothing; the terrain is everything." Indeed, we are designed to coexist with bacteria and viruses, and this cohabitation is the essence of our immune system and our life. Viruses are our parasites, and we are their hosts. An imbalance between the host and the parasite occurs, and the disease appears because of a deficient immune system.

Mesovaccination is the intradermal delivery of a vaccine. Even the famous Dr. Anthony Fauci wrote about the intradermal delivery of vaccines using small doses (La Montagne, 2004). Mesovaccination is already used for several vaccines—for example, the Bacille Calmette–Guérin (BCG) and smallpox vaccines are administered intradermally. The smallpox vaccine resulted in the worldwide elimination of this highly virulent disease, which is one of the triumphs of modern public health.

Compared with other delivery strategies, mesovaccination offers many advantages: small doses, reduced biohazard waste, decreased side effects, and pain-free vaccination. Intramuscular injection of a vaccine bypasses the skin's immune system (Egunsola, 2021; Kenney, 2004). The antigen of a vaccine triggers an immune response. When it's delivered to muscle tissue, it's thought to be

The Five Foundations of Percutaneous Hydrotomy

picked up by transient antigen-presenting cells or circulated to the lymph node. By contrast, intradermal injection of a vaccine delivers antigen directly into the skin, an anatomical space that contains large numbers of immune antigen-presenting cells and thus has the potential for greater immunogenicity than an intramuscular injection. Intradermally delivered vaccines may improve immunogenicity (Marra, 2013; Song, 2013).

One study showed that one-fifth of the standard influenza vaccine dose was sufficient six months after mesovaccination in adults (Kenney, 2004). The dose of the influenza vaccine was standardized to 15 micrograms (μg) in the early 1980s. Many studies have found no difference between the different intradermal influenza vaccine doses and the standard 15μg intramuscular influenza vaccine dose (Song, 2013). Research in this area is ongoing, and some are even doing research employing intradermal delivery of mRNA vaccines.

We aren't acting on the most extensive immune system—the skin. Viruses first enter through the oral, nasal, and lacrimal mucous membranes (Freitas Santoro, 2021). By stimulating the local immune barriers in the sinus as a preventive measure, it's possible to neutralize the viruses by the local cellular immune system, thus decreasing the viral load and preventing the spread of the virus into our bodies. Strengthening the immune system is vital for at-risk populations, such as the elderly, diabetics, the obese, and the immune-compromised.

The Energy Unit

This unit of competency is about how our cells store, produce, and use energy through the formation of adenosine triphosphate (ATP), the fundamental energy currency for all life. As we will see, it all goes back to water. ATP drives every aspect of cell function, and without it we would die within seconds. Animals store the energy obtained from the breakdown of food in ATP molecules; plants capture and store the energy they derive from light during photosynthesis in ATP molecules. Our nervous systems require enormous amounts of ATP. The dysfunction in cellular energy encompasses every physiological process. Albert Szent-Györgyi wrote that in every culture and every medical tradition before ours, healing was accomplished by moving energy (Szent-Györgyi, 1972).

Diseases like fibromyalgia, vertigo, tinnitus, heart palpitations, IBS, eating disorders, insomnia, depressive disorders, and many more are all consequences of diminished cellular energy. Treatment from a percutaneous hydrotomy perspective would include a cellular energy protocol, including the use of B vitamins, amino acids, magnesium, lithium, trace minerals, and local anesthetics. Methylene blue can also be used as a medication to increase the oxygen-carrying capacity of red blood cells as well as stimulate the mitochondria to optimize the production of ATP.

What Adenosine Triphosphate (ATP) Does

ATP is called the energy molecule. It is our energy currency that fuels our bodies; without it we would die in about seven seconds (Pollack, 2013). Inside the mitochondria, a process called oxidative

The Five Foundations of Percutaneous Hydrotomy

> phosphorylation generates thirty-six ATP molecules for each glucose molecule under normal conditions. ATP doesn't directly produce energy; rather, it stores energy and releases heat in biological systems. Specifically, ATP binds to the end of proteins inside the cell, causing them to unfold, which allows them to bind to the water inside the cells. We know that intracellular water is structured, meaning it's not a liquid, gas, or solid, but more like a gel. It's also essential to consider that structured water gives energy to the body. Without ATP, structured water doesn't form, and cell function ceases. In damaged mitochondria, ATP production is insufficient. For example, cancer cells hijack the cells and force the mitochondria to produce only 2 ATP per molecule of glucose, which is one of the primary hallmarks of the cancer process. As we will see in chapter 5, water has an abundance of energy from the electrons it holds due to the high electronegativity of the oxygen atoms (Pollack, 2013).

As mentioned above, the autonomic nervous system (ANS) stems from the vagus nerve and the nerves exiting the spinal cord, which control the body's automatic functions. It contains about 100 to 500 million neurons and has been described as the second brain or "brain within the gut" (Breit, 2018).

The ANS, specifically the sympathetic and parasympathetic nerves, governs the body's unconscious functions—"rest and digest" or "fight or flight." In today's fast-paced and demanding society, chronic stress has become commonplace. In modern times, our fight-or-flight system is needlessly activated through social media pressures, work-related stress, long and congested commutes, health and wellness concerns, family and relationship challenges, and societal issues. ANS dysfunction directly affects our energetic unit and results in disorders of the mind and the body such as insomnia, depression, muscle spasms, anxiety, pain syndromes, and IBS.

Prolonged ANS imbalances lead to neuroendocrine (e.g., thyroid disorders) or neuro-immune disorders (e.g., rheumatoid arthritis). These abnormalities don't always appear on biological examinations or medical imaging, hence the difficulties in managing these disorders using conventional medicine.

Percutaneous hydrotomy allows us to influence the ANS by placing certain products at the corresponding levels of the ANS. For example, injecting the areas of the cervical and thoracic spine levels can help control migraine headaches.

The treatment of the energy unit in percutaneous hydrotomy includes:

- Local anesthetics
- Trace elements and magnesium, potassium, and lithium
- Microdoses of antidepressants, at the level of energy points or along the spine

Percutaneous hydrotomy permits the restoration of cellular energy. Inside our cells, energy is provided by the Krebs cycle and mitochondrial respiration, which produces ATP. The restoration of intracellular enzymatic reactions can only occur with the proper nutrients and cofactors that drive normal cellular function. Water is essential for these cellular changes.

To summarize, percutaneous hydrotomy is involved in several mechanisms: cellular hydration with water, molecular water exchange, delivery of micronutrition to the cells, increase in

The Five Foundations of Percutaneous Hydrotomy

microcirculation, cellular regeneration, immune stimulation, cellular detoxification, and reestablishing homeostasis by increasing cellular senescence. In chapter 5, we will explore the physiologic basis of percutaneous hydrotomy, the role of water, and the biological terrain.

CHAPTER 5

How Percutaneous Hydrotomy Works and Its Physiologic Basis

Water is life's matter and matrix, mother and medium. There is no life without water.

— *Albert Szent-Györgyi*

The practice of percutaneous hydrotomy is an area of medicine that attempts to reevaluate our approach to chronic pain. It's no longer sufficient to base medical treatments solely on allopathic principles using drugs, radiation, or surgery. Understanding the physiology of water and the biological terrain is essential to grasp why percutaneous hydrotomy can heal chronic diseases.

The physiologic basis of percutaneous hydrotomy involves the natural body processes that are involved in maintaining function.

How Percutaneous Hydrotomy Works

For example, imagine that you've just sprained your ankle in a basketball game. The injury is physiologic because the body responds naturally to protect and heal the injured area. Inflammation, pain, heat, and swelling occur due to the movement of water and an increase in blood flow. The ankle is painful because the body releases chemicals that stimulate nerve endings, signaling the brain to rest the injured ankle and not walk. Again, the body is designed to protect and repair itself.

The essence of a human being is water—life begins and ends with it. Water is life's mater and matrix, mother and medium (Szent-Györgyi, 1972). Water is fascinating yet poorly understood, despite its colossal impact on human health. For example, why do diseased cells contain less water than healthy cells? Why is the water inside our cells structured like a gel rather than like a liquid? When we drink water, how does it assimilate into our cells? When a person fractures their ankle, it swells to twice its average size within minutes. How does water rush so quickly into the wound? Why is it impossible to aspirate the water with a needle? Unraveling the behavior of water at the molecular level is critical for determining how chronic diseases affect us.

Life originated in the oceans, and ironically, amniotic fluid is similar in composition to seawater, as René Quinton observed in the 1900s (Quinton, 1912). Water is the most extraordinary of substances. Our very existence depends on water and is simultaneously threatened by its scarcity. Humans survive mere days without water. Our blood's salt and mineral concentrations still reflect that of the primordial oceans. Remarkably, we've maintained these concentrations, while the oceans have since changed.

Understanding the water inside our cells helps us to envision how percutaneous hydrotomy helps. A human-fertilized egg (cell)

Stopping Pain

is over 90 percent water; a newborn is around 75 percent water; an infant is 70 percent water one year after birth; healthy adults maintain around 70 percent water, and it drops to 55 percent in the elderly (Jequier, 2010; Hall, 2015). Humans regulate water balance with precision; even a loss of 1 percent of body water is compensated for within twenty-four hours (Jequier, 2010).

Water supports connective tissues, forming a kind of hammock. The vital organs—the brain, lungs, heart, liver, and kidneys—contain the most water, which is between 60 percent and 80 percent. Even the water in bones, cartilage, intervertebral discs, and joints are precisely regulated (Lorenzo, 2019). All organs obey the law of compliance, which is determined by their water content. For example, each night our liver shrinks to half their average size by displacing water from their tissues. In other words, the compliance of the organ is the elasticity of that organ, including the subcutaneous tissues. Optimal compliance depends on water content and water quality. The ability of subcutaneous tissue to expand to many times its normal volume and recover safely is greatly underappreciated by the medical community (Hanke, 2004). Our hope is that by highlighting the unique properties of the tumescent state of the subcutaneous tissues, this discussion will spark interest in fully realizing the therapeutic implications of percutaneous hydrotomy.

Water differs in healthy cells versus diseased cells. Chronic diseases result in part from dehydration and disruptions in water and electrolyte homeostasis. Water provides the matrix for biochemical processes and the structural and dynamic integrity of cells. Dehydration is a sign of aging and chronic disease, affecting every bodily structure. For example, water accounts for 75 percent of brain mass (Zhang, 2018). In Parkinson's and Alzheimer's disease, MRI studies reveal that the hippocampus loses about 25 percent of its water content years before clinical signs are apparent (Qiu, 2022). Dehydrated or desiccated vertebral discs can't provide adequate space between the vertebrae, leading to nerve compression and pain. Tendons and ligaments become dehydrated with age, leading to a decrease in collagen and elasticity, which results in injuries.

Another vital example is how normal cells transition to cancer cells (Marques, 2021). How intracellular water moves in cancer cells versus healthy cells shows clear discrimination between them; the cancer cells display an enhanced mobility of intracellular water (Trouard, 2008; Morshita, 2019; Van Putten, 2021). Cancer cells divide and grow rapidly, so it makes sense that water must become more mobile and less structured to achieve this uncontrolled growth. Next, dysfunction appears with the drop in oxygenation: the cell will self-intoxicate to start a process of degeneration and finally die.

The Numerous Roles of Water

- Water serves multiple functions: a building material; a solvent, a reaction medium and reactant; a carrier for nutrients and waste products; in thermoregulation; and as a lubricant and shock absorber (Jequier, 2010).
- Water regulates vital biological processes including DNA transcription, protein synthesis, energy generation, cellular signaling, and neurotransmission.
- Water is a neutral polar inorganic compound that is a tasteless, odorless, and nearly colorless liquid with a hint of blue. Its structure is composed of two hydrogen atoms and one oxygen atom.

Stopping Pain

- Pure water has a pH of 7, which is neither acidic nor basic.
- Water is the universal solvent.
- Water covers 70.9 percent of the Earth's surface (Pollack, 2013).
- The Earth is a closed system, much like a terrarium, meaning it rarely loses or gains matter. The same water that existed on the Earth millions of years ago is still present today, and the water you drink contains the same molecules that dinosaurs drank (Sarafian, 2014).
- Nearly 97 percent of the world's water is salt water or otherwise undrinkable. Another 2 percent is packed in ice caps and glaciers, leaving 1 percent for all life-forms on Earth (Breedlove, 2018).
- Water regulates the Earth's temperature just as it regulates the body's temperature.
- Water is liquid at room temperature, while other similar molecules, like hydrogen and nitrogen, exist as a gas.
- The "stickiness" of water molecules holds them together at room temperature.
- All the water on Earth arrived by comets and asteroids billions of years ago.
- Hot water freezes faster than cold water, known as the Mpemba effect. It's unknown why this happens.
- Ice exhibits at least nineteen different phases with various crystalline structures (Gasser, 2021).

Structured Water or Exclusion Zone Water

We know that intracellular water possesses distinct properties different from bulk water and plays a fundamental role in normal cell activity. Basic chemistry teaches us that water traditionally exists

How Percutaneous Hydrotomy Works

in three states: liquid, gas, and solid. Dr. Gerald Pollack purports that a unique phase of water, called structured water, exists inside and outside the cells. This structured water is neither liquid, gas, nor solid, but rather "ordered" or "structured" and acts more like a gel. Dr. Pollack's book *The Fourth Phase of Water* describes how the water inside our cells as existing in a gelatinous form and refers to it as "exclusion zone" (EZ water for short). Exclusion zone water is so named because it excludes large solutes such as proteins. By excluding solutes, a charge separation occurs and forms an electrical potential in the cell, which is why it resembles a charged battery. The main point is that EZ water contains a lot of charges, and its character differs from that of bulk water (Pollack, 2014; Pollack, 2011).

Energy and Water

Water is the best conductor of energy and electricity in the body, fundamental to all life. Cells are composed of trillions of water molecules (octillions to be more precise), so small that if you counted every molecule in your body, 99 percent would be water molecules. Cells maintain a constant balance by releasing energy in many forms: optical, chemical, electrical, and mechanical. Consider that sunlight enters the capillaries and separates the charges forming EZ water. Water functions like a machine, converting radiant energy into mechanical energy. Photosynthesis is one such example, driving fluid upward against gravity in plant capillaries. The relevance here is how water relates to percutaneous hydrotomy, and how cellular health relies on the precise regulation of sodium and potassium across the cell membrane, maintaining an electrical charge gradient. Failure to maintain this balance results in cellular malfunction, disease, and death. Percutaneous hydrotomy helps restore and maintain that balance.

Nerves, Pain, and Anesthesia

We use many local anesthetics in percutaneous hydrotomy, so understanding their mechanism is useful. Imagine that you unexpectedly touch a hot stove. Reflexively, you withdraw your hand to avoid the unpleasant pain. Nerves mediate this withdrawal reflex by quickly signaling your brain to pull your hand back unconsciously. Noxious stimuli trigger nerve signals propagating to the brain, and nerves do this because they behave like a dischargeable battery. This charge separation is a central feature of nerve-signal transmission and is thought to result from ATP-driven sodium-potassium pumps. An alternative view suggests that the charge separation arises from EZ water. Support for this view is the following:

- Synthetic gels have significant negative potential, similar to cells. Yet there are no sodium-potassium pumps, nor membranes, at least in the way we think of cells.
- Local anesthetics prevent the brain from receiving the signal that a surgeon is making a skin incision. Anesthetics are said to block the sodium-potassium pump, interrupting the electrical conduction of the nerves and thus the charge separation.
- A recent discovery is that local anesthetics like lidocaine and bupivacaine profoundly affect intracellular water and diminish the amount of EZ water in the cells. The American chemist Linus Pauling suggested this many years ago (Kundacina, 2016). It will be interesting whether additional research confirms that the negative potential of the cell arises from the negative charge of EZ water or the sodium-potassium pumps, or perhaps some combination of both (Pollack, 2013).

Is the Heart Only a Pump?

The heart is an extraordinary organ, weighing about 300 grams, that circulates some 8,000 liters of blood per day at rest and much more during activity, never fatiguing. In terms of mechanical work, this equates to the heart lifting 100 pounds, one mile high. The heart performs an even more astonishing task of "pushing" blood, which is five times denser than water, through 60,000 miles of vessels with diameters often smaller than red blood cells, multiple times per minute. Such facts go beyond imagination.

A popular high school biology question is to trace the journey of a blood cell through the arteries, veins, and capillaries. Blood traveling from the heart exits through the large arteries, reaches the capillaries, then returns to the heart via the veins. The capillary system is massive, covering the equivalent of an entire football field. The purpose of blood circulation is to deliver oxygen to the cells and bring oxygen-poor blood and waste products back to the heart and the lungs for replenishment.

By examining the relative velocity of blood at various stages of circulation, we know blood moves the fastest in the large arteries and veins and the slowest in capillaries, similar to how water flows in a river. We know that the pressure at which blood is pumped from the heart doesn't explain capillary flow. The blood flow rate is nearly equal in both veins and arteries, meaning blood enters the heart just as quickly as it leaves. If a pump were present, blood would leave the heart faster than it entered, but that isn't the case. Physics alone can't explain blood circulation as it occurs in the human body. The red blood cells (6–7 microns) are larger than the capillaries (3–5 microns) and must contort as they pass—akin to pushing a partially deflated soccer ball through a drainpipe. Blood flow pauses in capillaries, which is necessary for the exchange of gases, nutrients, and waste products. So, if blood momentarily stops at the midpoint of its circular flow, and then starts moving again, what's the force behind blood movement as it makes its way back to the heart?

The answer may lie in the fact that water is a unique substance capable of holding energy. Since structured water releases energy, this could explain how blood drives through capillary beds and thus reflects more of a photosynthetic process than previously thought. Light is required to energize water, and thanks to our sun, plenty of light penetrates our bodies day and night to do the job (Pollack, 2013; Alexander, 2017; Marinelli, 2017; Mitchel, 2015).

How Water Functions as a Shock Absorber

Anatomically, bones normally press upon one another during deep knee bends or squats. But, despite the high forces placed upon joints, they move smoothly. This occurs because every joint is lined with cartilage to provide synovial fluid, collagen, hyaluronic acid, and proteoglycan (protein) subunits. The synovial fluid is 80 percent water and consists of highly charged polymers (Sophia-Fox, 2009), and hyaluronic acid strongly attracts water. If the protein surface becomes damaged, water will no longer protect it, leading to erosion, pain, and immobility—arthritis.

In the 1900s, Nobel laureate Albert Szent-Györgyi wrote about the possibility of water forming protective sheets, rubbing against one another, and acting as a lubricant for joint surfaces

How Percutaneous Hydrotomy Works

(Szent-Györgyi, 1972). Modern polymer research shows the effectiveness of water lubrication (Jahn, 2016). Common substances sliding past one another ordinarily have frictional coefficients of one. When hydrated, however, these polymeric surfaces have a frictional coefficient as low as 0.00001, which means that water reduces friction on the order of 100,000 times. Despite this research, the exact reasons for water's extraordinary lubrication capabilities remain obscure. One answer may lie within the positively charged water molecules (hydronium ions) lining the cartilage surfaces and repelling against each other (Pollack, 2013).

As cartilage ages, it becomes damaged, dehydrated, and inflamed (Sophia-Fox, 2009). People then resort to pain medications or having healthcare practitioners inject their arthritic joints with corticosteroids or hyaluronic acid to dull the pain. These healthcare providers are inadvertently performing percutaneous hydrotomy. Hyaluronic acid's principal action is its powerful hygroscopic (water-attracting) ability to absorb three hundred times its weight in water (Gupta, 2019). This localized increase of water in the joint helps with arthritis by creating an indirect tumescent state or hydrotomy cushion. Additionally, organic silicium, which is also used in percutaneous hydrotomy, has a high affinity for water and is crucial in bone metabolism (Reffitt, 2003).

Aging and arthritis always come back to water, and providing lubrication to arthritic joints is the key to healing the cells and decreasing the pain. These are reasons why we include water in percutaneous hydrotomy. However, these treatments no longer work when the damage is too extensive. Sometimes, other regenerative techniques like PRP or stem cells are required; other times, a total knee joint replacement is the only answer to stop the pain and to restore function.

The Idea of a Cellular Lavage

Percutaneous hydrotomy is an allopathic medical technique that differs in its mode of administration. It consists of injecting physiologic saline and other elements or subcutaneously, effectively creating a tumescent state or a hydrotomy cushion. The idea of using water in the form of saline to treat chronic diseases dates to the early 1900s. As previously referenced, René Quinton is credited with saving thousands of infants from disease, malnutrition, and dehydration by injecting them with plasma of Quinton, all before the time of intravenous lines and needles.

Arthritis becomes chronic when natural healing mechanisms go awry and become trapped in an imbalanced state. Flooding the arthritic joint with water will necessarily dilute the inflammatory and healing mediators. These pain mediators are flushed away through the systemic absorption of saline. When the tissue returns to its unexpanded state, the working point of the healing process will reset, which promotes healing (Koulakis, 2020). This hydrotomy cushion results in temporary swelling of the soft tissues, acting as a water reservoir that slowly releases medications and vitamins. A therapeutic lavage occurs when diseased tissue is exposed to ample amounts of physiologic water (saline); this is also referred to as a washout.

For many years, it was believed that the therapeutic effect of injecting solutions into the dermis or subcutaneous tissues was solely due to the pharmacological action of the injected drug. The available research suggests that drugs administered in the subcutaneous tissues allow longer pharmacological action or residence time in the area of the pain. Water plays a significant role in the pain response and participates in the beneficial effects of regenerative injection techniques. In addition, there's recent evidence that the skin harbors a network of glial cells within the nervous system, which can modulate pain. This could explain why treatments like mesotherapy and percutaneous hydrotomy yield promising results (Mammucari, 2020).

Several processes occur by placing water near the site of injury or disease:

- Water exchange can take place in the cells
- Water dilutes these painful neurotransmitters
- Delivery of minerals, vitamins, anti-inflammatories, and other medications produces a biologic effect
- Changes the chemical and physical properties of the inoculated solutions (e.g., osmolarity and pH)

Saline and the Placebo Effect

The impact of water is significant and more than previously believed. Biologists have always considered water a mere background carrier of the more essential molecules of life. Saline injections have traditionally served as placebo controls in research studies (Zhang, 2008).

A placebo, by definition, is a treatment that's designed to have no known therapeutic value. However, numerous studies show that saline injections have active analgesic effects (Altman, 2016). Dr. Roy Altman from the UCLA School of Medicine published a review study about the clinical benefit of saline injections for knee osteoarthritis. His team reviewed forty randomized controlled trials and concluded that saline isn't a placebo, but a treatment. They recommended that the pain relief associated with injecting saline should prompt healthcare providers to consider saline an additional treatment, not a placebo. A well-conducted study of sixty patients with moderate to severe pain after knee surgery showed that saline injections produced effective pain relief (Roseland, 2004).

In clinical practice, treatment should be directed toward maintaining normal balance. Percutaneous hydrotomy can address chronic diseases through several mechanisms and depart from the conventional "lock-and-key" interpretation of pathological states. The references suggesting that saline acts as a therapeutic modality and not a placebo are numerous (Zhang, 2008; Saltzman, 2017; Previtali, 2021; Gao, 2019; Acosta-Olivio, 2020; Linnanmäki, 2020; Simental-Mendía, 2020; Abate, 2018; Vora, 2012; Gazendam, 2021; Yeland, 2004).

A compelling example of percutaneous hydrotomy's benefits for back pain is its ability to rehydrate desiccated (dehydrated) vertebral discs. Diseased vertebral discs are associated with inflammation, dehydration, and nerve compression. Both discs and the cartilage have a strong, spongelike affinity for water (hydrophilic), a fact that is unfortunately neglected by many healthcare providers.

Cellular lavage in percutaneous hydrotomy, although not quite the same process used in surgery, is similar. In arthroscopic surgery, surgeons use saline to visualize the structures being operated on. The side effect of using saline in these surgeries is that the subcutaneous tissues absorb copious amounts of water. Indeed, surgeons have been performing percutaneous hydrotomy for a long time. Many studies in the surgery literature have shown that lavage alone is therapeutic (Yeh, 2020). This dilution of the intracellular water affects the chemical pain mediators (TNF, IL, bradykinins, histamines), promoting intracellular water exchange and normalizing acid-base balance. The dilution of cellular mediators has been referred to as the salting-in effect, which is the process of precipitation or separation of a substance from a solution.

Research shows that tumescent injections direct the expansion of subcutaneous tissue from the inside out, dilating the tissues. The interstitial tissue becomes saturated with fluid. The amount of time the saline stays in the tissues, or the fluid residence time, is normally about two to three hours. Systemic circulation eventually redistributes the fluid throughout the body and the injection site returns to normal. Although the spreading of medications and vitamins added to the saline requires study, general conclusions may be drawn regarding the expected dynamics of the additives (Koulakis, 2020).

Cellular regeneration requires water. The French word *refrachir* is appropriate in that we must change and *refresh* the water in the aquarium.

The Biological Terrain

Now, let's shift our focus to the concept of the *terrain*, which is the French word for soil. Just as soil is essential for plant growth, understanding the biological terrain is vital for comprehending how percutaneous hydrotomy benefits patients. Physiologist Claude Bernard taught that the internal environment or the body's "terrain" was more important than the pathogens that infected it.

Nearly two hundred years later, medical schools seldom teach about the principles of the biological terrain, leaving many health experts to ignore Bernard's wisdom, focusing solely on eradicating the ever-changing microorganisms (Bernard, 1859; Cody, 2018). For example, during the COVID-19 pandemic, public recommendations about strengthening our immune systems to protect us from pandemics were conspicuously absent. We possess tremendous abilities to strengthen our immune systems, which is essential for all infectious, autoimmune, and degenerative diseases. While COVID-19 led many to become paralyzed by fear, depending solely on pharmaceuticals and vaccines, others took it as a wake-up call to optimize their health and strengthen their biologic terrain.

It's crucial to highlight our chronic health problems related to nutrition. Each year, millions of tons of pesticides are dumped on our food, and our intestines react poorly to daily exposure to these pesticide-laden foods. Pathologies such as IBS result in the malabsorption of micronutrients (Kau, 2018). Our intestines function similarly to the Earth's topsoil. We should ask ourselves and one another: What does this do to our biological terrain and ecosystems? These processes interrupt our natural systems, causing the body to attack itself, as with autoimmune diseases. After years of these unnatural processes, our bodies become increasingly deregulated. Our biological terrain is in disarray, resulting in excessive incidents of chronic diseases, such as arthritis, Alzheimer's disease, diabetes, depression, dementia, and obesity. Acid-reducing drugs and proton pump inhibitors significantly affect the absorption of micronutrients from the gastrointestinal system (Hussain, 2021). Many patients with chronic arthritis don't follow an optimal diet or absorb adequate nutrients to correct their pathologies. An excellent example is chronic osteoporosis and the intestinal absorption of vitamin D and vitamin K2 (Capozzi, 2020). It should seem intuitive that the delivery of vitamins using percutaneous hydrotomy can help by bypassing the gastrointestinal tract.

How Percutaneous Hydrotomy Works

The Importance of the Biological Terrain or the Internal Milieu

French physiologist Claude Bernard was credited with the 160-year-old theory that the health of the "internal milieu" protects us from microbes such as bacteria and viruses (Bernard, 1859). He wrote, "The stability of the internal environment is the condition for the free and independent life." This is the underlying principle of what would later be called homeostasis (a term coined by Dr. Walter Cannon). Bernard taught that the terrain of the human body was more important than the pathogens that infect it. The internal milieu is the interstitial fluid that bathes and nourishes cells.

Around the same time as Bernard, Dr. Louis Pasteur, a chemist, gave a lecture about the specific role of microorganisms in metabolic processes, stating that we are surrounded by and harbor microorganisms in our bodies, which he called the germ theory (Manchester, 2007). He purported that when we are exposed to pathogens, we become ill if deficiencies or toxicities weaken our defenses.

Antoine Béchamp, also a chemist, had already established his terrain theory before Pasteur (Manchester, 2001). The two chemists apparently despised one another, even though both independently made similar discoveries. Imbalances in the cellular environment affect the entire organism, including the immune system. Béchamp argued that over time, a compromised immune system has difficulty fighting disease and maintaining health. This theory later evolved into what is now known as the biological terrain concept. The biological terrain consists of cells and the nutrient-filled fluid matrix that surrounds them. This specialized environment precisely regulates the intake of electrolytes, vitamins, minerals, and fluids, thereby nourishing all cells.

Stopping Pain

The argument of what's more important, the terrain or the pathogen, is circular in nature. One can go on to say, what is the molecule or the atom? The cells or the organs? The bacteria or the organism? One can't function without the other. For example, molecules are composed of atoms, but molecules are more stable than atoms. The organism needs both to survive; one isn't more important than the other. Our modern diseases haven't arrived by chance. Neither Béchamp nor Pasteur could have predicted that we would fabricate highly pathogenic viruses and bacteria in laboratories. Gain-of-function research has produced viruses never intended by nature. Antibiotic-resistant bacterial infections could have never happened before the invention of antibiotics.

No credible scientist questions the validity of the germ theory. Modern medicine was developed to focus on killing the pathogen, and it has worked against many pathological infections such as pneumonia and sepsis. Returning to the question: Which is more important, the biological terrain or eradicating the microbes? Again, the answer is that we need both. Modern lifestyles have degraded our biological terrain, resulting in manufactured diseases like diabetes, chronic obstructive pulmonary disease, and obesity. We can all be thankful that modern medicine has given us a way to combat deadly pathogens. Béchamp gave legitimacy to the idea that strengthening our biological terrain undeniably helps our natural defense systems to fight chronic diseases (Whitcomb, 2022). Unlike the germ theory, the terrain theory helps explain why some people get sick while others don't when exposed to the same pathogens.

Pasteur initially opposed the idea of the internal milieu, and he believed that microbes outside of the body, such as bacteria and viruses, caused most illnesses and diseases. However, shortly before Pasteur's death, he was quoted as claiming that the "Milieu Interior"

How Percutaneous Hydrotomy Works

theory (proposed by Drs. Bernard and Béchamp at the time) was correct, that illness and disease are caused primarily by imbalances in the body's biological terrain. Pasteur said, "The microbe is nothing; the terrain is everything."

Other scientists also believed in Bernard's internal milieu hypothesis (Manchester, 2007; Schultz, 2008). A quote from Dr. Rudolph Virchow, the so-called "father of modern pathology," supports this idea: "If I could live my life over again, I would devote it to proving that germs seek their natural habitat—diseased tissue—rather than being the cause of dead tissue. In other words, mosquitoes seek the stagnant water but do not cause the pool to become stagnant." The symptoms of flu or pneumonia (fever, chills, cough, and excess mucus production) are secondary illnesses; the first "illness" is a loss of health in the underlying tissues. The better solution is to optimize our internal milieu and use medicines only when necessary.

Every living organism comes equipped with its janitorial service that goes to work when the cell dies. The vital force programs them to clean up the substances that are no longer vital. As contrary as it seems, germs are attracted to diseased tissues and are not the primary cause of it. The importance of water in healing chronic diseases can't be understated, yet it's often overlooked and misunderstood by healthcare providers (Cody, 2018). Every percutaneous hydrotomy protocol utilizes water because regeneration of our biologic terrain can't take place without it. The next chapter delves into the protocols of percutaneous hydrotomy used in clinics called mesochelation, mesoperfusion, and mesovaccination.

CHAPTER 6

The Fundamental Techniques of Percutaneous Hydrotomy

By now, you should understand what percutaneous hydrotomy is, how it was developed, the products used, and that it treats chronic diseases and pain. To summarize, it is a nonsurgical regenerative technique performed in a clinic or hospital that introduces a hydrotomy solution via injection or infusion around painful areas. The hydrotomy solution promotes the milieu supporting the healing of cells and tissues using physiologic saline, medications, and minerals.

Percutaneous hydrotomy solutions contain saline, minerals, vitamins, amino acids, anti-inflammatories, and local anesthetics. Medications like corticosteroids, when indicated, are used in tiny dilute doses; the quantity of medicine is reduced on average by a factor of 1,000 compared to oral administration. By

The Fundamental Techniques of Percutaneous Hydrotomy

addressing the properties of the medications—the pH, viscosity, and osmolarity—percutaneous hydrotomy injections are well tolerated. The adverse effects of certain products can be decreased by delivering these products in diluted solutions. The dermatology literature has shown that intradermal injection of diluted corticosteroids is safe and effective (Luther, 2020); in percutaneous hydrotomy, corticosteroids are diluted at least ten times based on volume. Klein et al. found no adverse effect of tumescent antibiotics (cefazolin and metronidazole), lidocaine, epinephrine, nor saline. The subcutaneous injection of cefazolin and metronidazole is "off-label" according to the United States Food and Drug Administration–approved package insert labeling. Yet subcutaneous antibiotic delivery, as well as many other medications, are commonly utilized (Klein, 2017).

Percutaneous hydrotomy rebalances the tissues and relieves pain. This is the concept of complementary-regenerative medicine. Depending on the situation, other regenerative methods may be employed, such as platelet-rich plasma (PRP), prolotherapy, ultrasound, stem cells, red-light therapy, or hyperbaric oxygen treatments. The primary goal of percutaneous hydrotomy in chronic pain conditions is stimulating regenerative processes in the cells of ligaments, tendons, and joint capsules, thus restoring joint stability.

Mesochelation

Mesochelation is a technique, as its name suggests, that involves the skin, mesotherapy, and chelation. Chelation is the act of binding a chelating agent such as EDTA to metal ions and other molecules, which are then excreted from the body. *Meso* means the "middle" layer of the dermis or skin. Thus, mesochelation refers to mesotherapy and chelation to treat certain conditions.

Mesochelation is the preferred technique for treating osteoarthritis. After cleaning the skin aseptically, a tiny mesotherapy needle is used to inject saline and local anesthetic into the area of concern, improving patient comfort. Then a solution containing saline, EDTA, minerals, and anti-inflammatories is placed locally over the region so that they may act directly on the diseased cells. We always use EDTA in low doses to avoid the risk of pain on injection or other side effects (Guez, 2021).

We create a tumescent state or hydrotomy cushion, using physiologic saline to provide the area with targeted micronutrition (vitamins, anti-inflammatories, and trace minerals). Multiple treatments are often required, depending on the situation. The mesochelation technique helps most forms of arthritis, except for very advanced cases such as end-stage arthritis or hip osteoarthritis. Healthcare professionals are familiar with intravenous or intramuscular treatments, but few are trained in intradermal or subcutaneous treatments. Similarly, hypodermoclysis is rarely performed for therapeutic purposes and is often limited to its role in hydrating elderly patients (Giordano, 2018). However, subcutaneous techniques have the considerable advantage of being noninvasive. The hydrotomy cushion forms under the skin, and the short mesotherapy needle can't hit deep organs or nerves. The mesochelation protocol is practiced safely.

Chelation and Ethyl-Diamino-Tetra-Acetate (EDTA)

EDTA is a synthetic amino acid and has a long history in medicine (George, 2021). It's widely used to sequester divalent and trivalent metal and mineral ions (lead, mercury, arsenic, aluminum, cobalt, calcium). EDTA is used in chelation therapy for lead, mercury, and heavy metal poisoning; coronary heart disease; calcifications (osteophytes), and arthritis (Cacchio, 2009; Sears, 2013).

The Fundamental Techniques of Percutaneous Hydrotomy

EDTA acts to mobilize calcifications in the bones, tendons, and ligaments. Understanding calcium transport is paramount to understanding how chronic diseases come about. Calcification is a phenomenon often regarded by pathologists as evidence of cartilage disease and cell death (Menkes, 2004; Kim, 1995; Boraldi, 2021). For example, sciatica is nerve pain resulting from compression by osteophytes, which can be clearly seen on X-rays. Lumbar canal stenosis is a common cause of back pain where there is thickening and calcium deposition in the ligament structures themselves. Removing the diseased calcium can reduce the mechanical pressure created by vertebral osteophytes. Calcific tendinitis of the shoulder is the pathological buildup of calcium in the tendons, causing pain; the mesochelation protocol utilizes EDTA to treat calcific tendinitis of the shoulder by displacing the pathological calcium (Cacchio, 2009). EDTA mobilizes and chelates the diseased calcium, which ends up in circulation and is excreted in the urine (Sears 2013; George, 2021).

Figure. Mesochelation treatment of the shoulder calcific tendonitis (frozen shoulder) before and after a series of percutaneous hydrotomy treatments.

Mesoperfusion

This technique uses the therapeutic properties of mesochelation but takes the form of a subcutaneous infusion. The mesoperfusion technique utilizes anywhere from one to twenty-four outlets (sometimes called "the octopus") to deliver the hydrotomy solution (Guez, 2021). Mesoperfusion is most often performed on chronic diseases of the lower back and the knees.

Many ask how cortisone steroid shots differ from percutaneous hydrotomy. Cortisone injections are often performed under sedation, use X-ray guidance, treat one or two intervertebral spaces, and use high doses of corticosteroids. Percutaneous hydrotomy protocols use dilute doses of corticosteroids placed subcutaneously, and not every protocol uses corticosteroids. Furthermore, neither X-rays nor sedation are necessary.

Several studies have highlighted the use of mesochelation and mesoperfusion in treating patients with back pain (Nguyen, 2009; Guez, 2021; Constantino, 2011; Guez, 1998; Vidal, 2019). Dr. Guez conducted a study involving twenty-five patients with back pain, utilizing mesoperfusion as a treatment method. To assess the treatment's effectiveness, patients' pain levels were measured using the Visual Analog Scale (VAS). At the start of the study, the average pre-treatment VAS score was 7.2/10. After 3.5 months of mesoperfusion treatments, the average VAS score significantly decreased to 1.8/10. These findings suggest that mesoperfusion positively impacts the reduction of lumbar back pain. These results align with our clinical observations and numerous patient testimonies presented in chapter 9. However, it's important to interpret these findings within the context of further research, recognizing that percutaneous hydrotomy is not a panacea but rather one treatment option within the complex landscape of chronic back pain management.

Dr. Guez has presented the results of his practice and studies on percutaneous hydrotomy at various international conferences, including Strasbourg, France, at the 5th National Congress of Mesotherapy (2007); Mexico, at the 12th Congress of Mesotherapy (2008); Munich, Germany, at the German Society of Mesotherapy (2009); Moscow, Russia, at the 13th International Congress of Mesotherapy (2011); and Tunisia, at the 15th International Congress

The Fundamental Techniques of Percutaneous Hydrotomy

of Mesotherapy (2019). Additionally, Guez (2019) was presented at the 50th Annual Regional Anesthesiology and Acute Pain Medicine Meeting in Orlando, Florida (2025).

Mesovaccination

Mesovaccination has already been discussed in chapter 4. In summary, it is a method of placing a dilute amount of a subdermal vaccine to educate the skin's immune system. It's important to dissociate the so-called "classic" vaccination from mesovaccination. The concept of vaccination is fundamental to the treatment and the prevention of certain chronic inflammatory diseases. It's the mode of administration of vaccines in excessive quantities and far from their site of action that is questionable. With mesovaccination, the protocol is different, and with intradermal administration, the skin makes up a barrier immune filter. Undesirable side effects are minimal because the vaccines (influenza, pneumococcal, anti-Haemophilus, or polyvalent) are diluted by one thousand times compared to conventional vaccines. This effect has been confirmed with the immunologic effect of intradermal tetanus toxin administration (Pitzurra, 1981).

As previously mentioned, we have two types of immunity: (1) humoral (circulating in the blood) and (2) cellular. Intradermal and targeted mesovaccination allow better stimulation of the immune defenses. The skin is the gateway to the fundamental unit of competence.

After numbing the skin with an anesthetic cream or ice, a healthcare provider will perform multiple intradermal injections with diluted doses of vaccines, making it possible to stimulate local immune defenses. The immunogenicity of the skin is the ability to trigger an immune response and produce antibodies in large numbers. The skin's immune reservoir is poorly exploited by healthcare providers, including dermatologists.

After the treatment sessions, we often see the "rebound effect" (or paradoxical effect), corresponding to an "awakening" of the antibodies, which lasts for about twenty-four to forty-eight hours. This sign is very positive, as it means the body is reacting to the treatment. The rebound effect will be less apparent over subsequent sessions. When the rebound effect completely disappears, the education of antibodies is finished, and the patient has recovered.

The Actions of Percutaneous Hydrotomy

Various diseases have specific causes and symptoms. Local treatment can act directly on the lesion. For example, knee osteoarthritis is a disease localized to the knee cartilage or to the bone cells (chondrocytes). Local healing and regeneration can occur by delivering the treatment directly to the knee instead of orally or intravenously.

To review, percutaneous hydrotomy acts on the five competency units by applying the following mechanisms:

- Extracellular hydration with a physiological saline solution
- Water as the vehicle of the therapeutic products
- Delivery of cellular micronutrition via injectable trace elements, vitamins, magnesium, organic silicium, and amino acids
- Increase in microcirculation by vasodilators and antiplatelet agents
- Immune stimulation (mesovaccination): injections without product or addition of tiny doses of dilute vaccines

The Fundamental Techniques of Percutaneous Hydrotomy

- Improvement of cellular balance
- Cellular detoxification of heavy metals and calcium with the technique of mesochelation

Undesirable Effects and Precautions

The side effects of percutaneous hydrotomy are rare; it has an excellent safety history. All regenerative techniques involve the delivery of a solution using a needle. Percutaneous hydrotomy is the delivery of fluids via a tiny needle resulting in an augmentation of volume in the subcutaneous space. All injections carry inherent risk; therefore, an aseptic technique is essential. In France, Dr. Guez's clinic has never had a serious side effect in over forty years of giving these injections (Guez, 2021). It's because Dr. Guez uses excellent technique and adheres to his protocols.

The correct steps for performing a safe and aseptic procedure are as follows:

- Wear disposable gloves.
- Prepare single-use needles and syringes.
- Prep the area with an appropriate disinfectant.
- Warn the patient that a specific area will be treated and have them in a comfortable position (supine if necessary).
- Prepare the drugs to be injected.
- Carefully clean the area of the skin to be treated.
- Inject the solution into the selected points.
- Wait a few minutes before allowing the patient to stand up again.
- Dispose of medical waste in an appropriate container.
- Complete the medical record as necessary.

Stopping Pain

Several side effects of mesotherapy have been documented. Most of these cases are related to the administration of deoxycholic acid for weight loss and cosmetic procedures. Some of the adverse events reported are bruising and edema due to the chemicals used, skin necrosis, bacterial infections, allergic reactions, skin atrophy, granulomas, and vagal syndromes (Sarkar, 2011; Sivagnanam, 2019). Infection is usually from using a poor or incorrect aseptic technique.

Pain on injection occurs with certain therapeutics, such as EDTA, making the experience unpleasant. The importance of tumescent anesthesia with lidocaine and the proper dose of EDTA can't be underestimated. Mild transient pain after injection is normal and subsides quickly. Blanching and edema of the skin is common and occurs because of the volume in the subcutaneous tissue that resolves quickly. Some people feel mild pressure over the injection area, but this is temporary. It's important to remember that patients with nerve pain due to herniated discs experience increased skin sensitivity in the corresponding dermatomes, which are patches of skin wired to a single nerve in your spine. Injecting solutions that are hypertonic, meaning they have a higher concentration than our body fluids, can cause discomfort. To avoid these issues, it's common practice in percutaneous hydrotomy protocols to use isotonic solution for injections. Isotonic solutions have the same concentration as our body fluids, reducing the risk of pain or tissue damage upon injection. Secondary effects can result from the use of medications such as pentoxifylline, which may cause vasodilation (dilating of the blood vessels) and facial warming. Percutaneous hydrotomy should be used with caution in patients with bleeding or coagulation disorders.

The Fundamental Techniques of Percutaneous Hydrotomy

Percutaneous hydrotomy protocols are designed to decrease the patient's chances of having a painful experience. With chronic pain, we often observe an aggravation of the symptoms after the first percutaneous hydrotomy treatment. It often appears paradoxical, but Dr. Michel Pistor and others have described this phenomenon (Pistor, 1979). Subsequent treatments are better tolerated and provide relief in these types of patients.

Critical reviews of mesotherapy, prolotherapy, hypodermoclysis, and tumescent anesthesia support the safety of subcutaneous fluid administration (Pistor, 1979; Dalloz-Bourguignon, 1980). These techniques presented should only be performed by healthcare providers who have received proper training certified by the International Society for Percutaneous Hydrotomy (ISPH).

In the field of pain medicine, diverse invasive procedures are conducted for the purpose of diagnosis and pain relief. However, procedures conducted by inexperienced healthcare providers can increase the potential for complications. To prevent this, adequate training, a sound understanding of anatomy, and proper injection techniques are necessary.

We have learned about the principal techniques used in percutaneous hydrotomy and their applications. In the next chapter we will delve more into specific chronic diseases and how percutaneous hydrotomy can help.

CHAPTER 7

How Percutaneous Hydrotomy Treats Common Conditions

Man cannot become a competent surgeon without the full knowledge of human anatomy and physiology, and the physician without physiology and chemistry flounders along aimlessly, never able to gain any accurate conception of disease, practicing a sort of popgun pharmacy, hitting now the malady and again the patient, he himself not knowing which.
—Sir William Osler (1849–1919)

Sir William Osler expresses well the relationship between the basic sciences and clinical medicine. Indeed, since the Middle Ages, wise physicians have realized that human diseases are essentially disordered physiology. Pathophysiology is the convergence of

How Percutaneous Hydrotomy Treats Common Conditions

pathology with physiology associated with a disease or an injury. Therefore, with the knowledge of the structure and the function comes the ability to understand diseases and design effective treatments.

The relationship between pathology and physiology is a two-way street. Diseases are experiments of nature that uncover previously unknown or unappreciated physiologic mechanisms. If a bacterial organism triggers an illness, the body reacts with molecular and cellular responses that are the signs and the symptoms of the disease. Investigating these physiologic mechanisms advances our fundamental medical knowledge.

Within the context of percutaneous hydrotomy, we have a platform to treat chronic disease conditions by taking advantage of the body's biological terrain. Claude Bernard and others emphasized that treating the body's biological terrain, not just the symptoms, is the key to healing. Since the basis of percutaneous hydrotomy involves subcutaneous injections, an understanding of the skin is essential. We access these interconnected systems (the immune system, the cardiovascular system, the nervous system, the gastrointestinal system, the musculoskeletal system) through the skin and the subcutaneous tissues. Everything affects the biological terrain including diet, habitation, relationships, emotions, thoughts, lifestyle, and genes.

Integrative medicine draws upon complementary and allopathic medicine, applying a well-combined approach. Individualization is the future of medicine—what works for one may not work for another. Just because a celebrity has endorsed a supplement or your friend lost weight eating a particular diet doesn't mean it works for everyone. People who follow the latest fad diet, health trend, or supplement are hoping for miracles.

Stopping Pain

Healing is an inside job that requires time and investment by both the patient and the practitioner. Chronic diseases are never resolved with a quick fix—they take years to develop and can take years to heal. Balancing the biological terrain is a good first step since diseases develop as a result of a depleted terrain. The importance of water can't be overemphasized. Water is the aquarium for the salts that assure cellular function, giving us life energy.

Chronic diseases and pain affect millions worldwide, with conditions like back pain tripling over the last forty years; it has been labeled the disease of the century and imposes more disability than any other disease or injury (Volinn, 2022). Musculoskeletal conditions are a significant cause of years lived with disability worldwide. Pain is why patients seek medical care. The patients' pain persists; even worse, the patient merely exists in a vicious cycle of taking medications. Modern healthcare inadequately addresses chronic pain, and many suffer needlessly, often until death.

Percutaneous hydrotomy proceeds differently. It can be applied to a range of conditions and injuries:

- Osteoarthritis in the neck, shoulder, spine, knees, hands, and feet
- Narrow lumbar canal, sciatica, neuralgia, herniated disc
- Bone spurs (osteophytes) with mechanical compression
- Rheumatoid arthritis and autoimmune diseases
- Psoriatic arthritis

Musculoskeletal injuries arise from factors like trauma, aging, poor nutrition, inflammation, and insulin resistance. At their core, musculoskeletal injuries are a malfunction of the fundamental unit. These problems can occur during violent sports efforts, friction

How Percutaneous Hydrotomy Treats Common Conditions

against calcifications of bone, or trauma. The discomfort can persist for months and sometimes for years. Conventional medicine employs rest, taping, elevation, ice, and analgesics. All too often, patients and healthcare providers rely on surgery as the solution. Indeed, severe injuries and trauma requiring hospitalization aren't amenable to percutaneous hydrotomy.

Migraines

Severe migraines are described as the worst conceivable pain, and many describe the experience as "hell on earth" as it grows, causing a full-body malaise and being bedridden wearing an eye mask for days. Some even contemplate suicide.

Migraines are among the top ten global causes of years lived with disability (Vos, 2015). For millions, migraines are leading causes of emergency room visits (Tepper, 2008; Burch, 2015). The genesis of headaches involves dysfunction of energetic, neuromuscular, and circulatory systems, which results from anxiety, stress, depression, and insomnia. Symptoms are treated with pharmacological oral agents such as anti-inflammatories, narcotics, antihistamines, and injections such as steroids, triptans, and Botox (Tepper, 2008; Ramachandran, 2014). Still, these agents never address the root cause of the problem. The fundamental problem revolves around the neurological and circulatory units of competency.

The underlying causes of migraines are complex and multifactorial. According to the work of French physician Robert Maigne, 80 percent of migraines are of cervical (neck) origin (Meloche,1993). He performed painstaking dissections in thirty cadavers to elucidate the anatomy of the superficial nerves of the neck and back; his work shows that these superficial nerves are the pain generators and ignored by healthcare providers. Another type, vascular migraines, are extremely difficult to treat and diagnose.

Migraines often arise from muscle spasms secondary to nerve irritation. For example, the cervical root of the trigeminal nerve can be compressed by osteophytes at the C2 vertebrae. Osteophytes are hypercalcified deformations and can often be felt on examination. In our experience, many C2 vertebral deformities result from accidents, head trauma (whiplash), or patients sleeping on their stomachs with the neck in extension. Arnold's neuralgia is another type of migraine caused by injury or irritation of the occipital nerves, which travel from the base of the skull through the scalp.

Percutaneous hydrotomy can successfully treat migraines. French physician Dr. Yannick Lemaire studied the treatment of migraines using percutaneous hydrotomy (Lemaire, 2016). From a healing standpoint, it's essential to treat the energy system of the cells. By injecting saline, minerals, vitamins, anti-inflammatories, magnesium, and local anesthetics, we can address the root cause or etiology of migraines. For example, riboflavin (vitamin B2) is central to energy metabolism.

The injection depth is only half a millimeter (about the length of a single grain of rice), which is consistent with large dilution mesotherapy techniques and reaches the superficial nerves under the skin (Lemaire, 2016). In this sense, this treatment is similar to local anesthetic blocks, mesotherapy, or perineural superficial injections (Akbas, 2021; Caputi, 1997; Levin, 2010; Linetsky, 2004). Migraines require multiple treatments, and many of our patients have found long-term relief. Studies are ongoing evaluating the effect of saline injections for chronic migraines (Kim, 2019).

How Percutaneous Hydrotomy Treats Common Conditions

Clinical Case: Madame S., fifty-four years old

Migraines

Before the percutaneous hydrotomy treatments, I suffered severe migraines, cervical tension, and malaise. I tried several medications (muscle relaxants and anti-inflammatories), physiotherapy, and massage, but to no avail. I tried mesotherapy, which provided relief, but only for a short time. And then I heard about percutaneous hydrotomy. I thought, why not give it a try when you don't know where to turn. And there it was a miracle! After six weeks (one session per week), I was completely free of migraines and neck pain. I encourage people with migraine and neck issues to try percutaneous hydrotomy.

Clinical case: Mr. S., forty-nine years old

Migraines

Mr. S. presented with a twenty-year history of chronic migraines. He has undergone multiple studies and his headaches were labeled idiopathic, which is a basket term in medicine meaning the healthcare provider doesn't know the cause. MRIs, X-rays, and lab tests were all negative. The headaches would last twenty-four to forty-eight hours, leaving him incapacitated and unable to work or ride bicycles, his favorite hobby. We started treatment using the hand-syringe mesochelation technique to reduce the diseased calcium of the osteophytes, which were likely compressing the nerves.

> He gradually experienced the disappearance of his migraines. Since starting percutaneous hydrotomy treatments, he says that his life is amazing, because nothing else ever touched the migraines. He recently needed another treatment when he felt a migraine coming on right before a seven-day cycling event across the state of Iowa, which he completed with no problems.

Temporomandibular Joint Syndrome

Temporomandibular joint syndrome (TMJ) is a common disorder affecting the jaw and the surrounding joints, muscles, and ligaments. TMJ is akin to osteoarthritis of the jaw and results from trauma, an improper bite, arthritis, and degeneration of the C2–C3 intervertebral discs. Facial pain, jaw cracking, headaches, difficulty in mouth opening, and bruxism (clenching of the jaw at night) are typical symptoms of TMJ.

TMJ often follows psychological and emotional trauma presenting with psychological symptoms: stress, anxiety, sleep disorders, depression, spasms, and eating disorders (Li, 2021). The body's autonomic nervous system is overstimulated, as if the energy developed to adapt to the external environment remains blocked inside. This self-destructive system triggers neuroendocrine, neurohormonal, and neuroimmune dysfunctions. Patients experience a weakening of the organism, lack of energy, and inability to accomplish tasks, as well as dizziness, palpitations, and irritable bowel syndrome. Healthcare providers often treat patients with antidepressants, muscle relaxants, analgesics, and sleeping pills. In conventional dentistry, a restrictive mouthpiece is prescribed.

How Percutaneous Hydrotomy Treats Common Conditions

The alternative in percutaneous hydrotomy for TMJ syndrome is to treat the fundamental, neurological, and energetic competency units. The mesochelation technique provides hydration and reduces diseased calcium in the joints, helping to restore function to vertebral discs and cartilage while optimizing cellular metabolism.

The benefits of lavage in TMJ are well known (Li, 2021). A clinic utilizing mesotherapy techniques on TMJ studied the effects of a combination of an NSAID, local anesthetic, and pentoxifylline every two weeks (Andre, 2015); all patients except one found relief from their TMJ pain. We've found that amino acids have a dynamic effect, improving joint plasticity and the possibility of eliminating pain and cracking. Percutaneous hydrotomy employs energy therapies based on mesotherapy principles called a mesostress protocol (Guez, 2021). It's performed on specific points taken from Chinese medicine, such as the temples, thyroid, stomach, and heart regions.

A TMJ protocol would include weekly injections of EDTA, procaine (vasodilator), magnesium, trace elements, and tiny amounts of antidepressants. This treatment alleviates the need for drugs such as Xanax. Many patients experience dramatic improvements from the first or the second session.

The Shoulder

The shoulder is the third most commonly injured joint, after the knee and the ankle (Luime, 2004). Shoulder injuries result from trauma or repetitive overuse, often from overhead activities. The shoulder is highly mobile because of the minimal containment of the humeral head, but the trade-off for this mobility is decreased stability, making the shoulder prone to various types of injuries.

One such condition is called adhesive capsulitis, better known as frozen shoulder. In 1872, Dr. Simon Duplay described it as a

Stopping Pain

relentless painful peri-arthritic condition characterized by shoulder pain, especially at night, and decreased movement (Noel, 2000; Bunker, 2011). Surprisingly (or not), it primarily affects middle-aged sedentary people. Conventional treatment is typically conservative and includes NSAIDs and analgesics, exercise, and therapeutic ultrasound (Manske, 2008, Ramirez, 2019).

Despite the term "frozen," the tendon calcifications aren't hard and crystallized—they have a toothpaste-like consistency. Calcium normally exists in bones and teeth, and when calcium deposits elsewhere, we call this pathologic calcification (kidney stones, calcium deposits in tendons, and osteophytes). Though poorly understood, frozen shoulder is caused by inflammation, excess vitamin D, and injuries (Ramirez, 2019; DeCarli, 2014).

In a randomized controlled study, Italian researchers used mesotherapy to inject a dilute solution of EDTA (1 ml), procaine (2 ml), and saline (3 ml) subcutaneously into the shoulders of eighty patients with frozen shoulder over three to six sessions (Cacchio, 2009). Amazingly, 62.5 percent of the calcifications completely disappeared on X-ray after four weeks, significantly improving pain and shoulder function. Another Italian paper recently reported complete pain resolution in twenty-nine out of thirty-one patients with frozen shoulder using a similar protocol (Mammucari, 2020). A study published by the American College of Rheumatology showed that the abnormal shoulder calcifications had entirely disappeared in nearly two-thirds of the patients after four weeks using saline, a local anesthetic, EDTA, and magnesium without any adverse effects (Cacchio, 2009). Another Italian group used mesotherapy to treat frozen shoulder using saline, EDTA, and lidocaine. Over 90 percent of the patients had an improvement in their VAS pain score, and

How Percutaneous Hydrotomy Treats Common Conditions

80 percent had complete disappearance of the abnormal calcium (Soncini, 1998).

The alternative in percutaneous hydrotomy is using mesochelation and vasoactive treatments to unblock the capsule, remove the calcium, decrease pain, and increase joint mobility. So, what's the difference between percutaneous hydrotomy and mesotherapy in the case of a frozen shoulder? They are similar, except that more saline is used in percutaneous hydrotomy. The mesochelation protocol calls for saline, EDTA, procaine, magnesium, vasodilators, B vitamins, and anti-inflammatories. Our experience in treating frozen shoulder is excellent, and most of the calcium deposits disappear.

Although the mechanism of sodium EDTA in calcific tendinitis is not fully understood, it's postulated that the action of EDTA is due to its chelating capacity (Cacchio, 2009). Sodium EDTA is a synthetic amino acid that directly acts on the excess calcium, which is the fundamental mechanism of how EDTA works to help arthritis. The rationale for its clinical use in calcific tendinitis of the shoulder is because disodium EDTA binds and removes the calcium deposits, which are then excreted in the urine. Percutaneous hydrotomy is a safe, simple, and effective treatment for shoulder calcific tendinitis. Usually, an average of six weekly sessions results in medium-term healing.

The Story of T.J. Dillashaw—UFC Athlete

T.J. Dillashaw is a well-known MMA fighter. His experience with percutaneous hydrotomy highlights how this innovative treatment can play a crucial role in the recovery of athletes. Dillashaw was training for a highly anticipated fight that would mark his comeback after a two-year hiatus. Six weeks before the fight, he sustained a left shoulder injury during training following an aggressive left hook. The mechanism of his injury was excessive lateral rotation, and his medical examination revealed a left rotator cuff injury. His pain at rest was about a 4/10 and 10/10 with activity. His pain improved with anti-inflammatory medications, rest, and massage, but regular physical activity was impossible. Dillashaw had had previous shoulder injuries and surgeries. He was determined to see if percutaneous hydrotomy could help his shoulder and allow him to fight. I explained that it would take several treatments, and a regenerative protocol was prescribed since we knew it was a tendon injury. Using a combination of physiologic saline, amino acids, fat-soluble vitamins, magnesium, pentoxifylline, procaine, trace minerals, local anesthetics, and anti-inflammatories, the hydrotomy cushion was placed around the areas of pain in his shoulder. Note that the anti-doping authorities were consulted about the percutaneous hydrotomy procedure, and the regulations were respected at all times concerning injections. After the first treatment, Dillashaw felt relief but was unable to train. Following the second treatment, he noted that his rehabilitation went much better and that with activity, his pain level was now a 7/10. The third treatment resulted in better function and lower pain levels. He received two more treatments, at which point his shoulder was essentially pain free. Already the percutaneous hydrotomy treatment was a success. The bout lasted five rounds, Dillashaw sustained multiple injuries to his knee and his face, and he won the fight in a decision. He acknowledged that percutaneous hydrotomy helped to save his fight (Edwards, 2021).

How Percutaneous Hydrotomy Treats Common Conditions

Osteoarthritis

Osteoarthritis (OA) is a painful condition involving degeneration of bone cartilage, affecting over 32 million people in the United States and worldwide (Cross, 2014; *Science Daily*, 2016). Hip and knee OA are leading causes of global disability. In percutaneous hydrotomy, osteoarthritis primarily involves the fundamental unit—the cells (Roush, 2002). We can apply this way of thinking to many conditions: skin wrinkles are analogous to arthritis of the skin; a cataract is analogous to arthritis of the eye; balance disorders such as tinnitus and hearing loss are forms of osteoarthritis of the auditory apparatus. Age is the strongest risk factor for osteoarthritis, but aging per se is not the cause.

Joint osteoarthritis is best understood as a disturbance of the balance between the synthesis and the degradation of cartilage. OA is caused by inflammatory diseases which can be traumatic, metabolic, infectious, crystal-induced, reactive, or autoimmune (Mobasheri, 2016); the inflammation cascade destroys the cartilage. Dehydration, degeneration, abnormal separation, and progressive cartilage loss are visible under a microscope, and its biomarkers are easily measured. Bone deformities, stiffness, decreased mobility, and pain are experienced every day. In chapter 5, Albert Szent-Györgyi described water forming protective sheets rubbing against one another and acting as a lubricant for joint surfaces.

Conventional medicine suggests weight reduction, using a cane, exercise, physical therapy, osteoarthritis supplements (e.g., glucosamine, chondroitin, turmeric), analgesics, antidepressants, NSAIDs, local anesthetics, hyaluronic acid, or epidural corticosteroid injections. These conservative treatments do help many people; however, none of these consider the root cause of arthritis. In case of failure, surgeons replace the joint with a prosthesis.

Stopping Pain

The alternative in percutaneous hydrotomy is utilizing the mesochelation and vasoactive protocols, which accomplishes:

- Hydration of the cartilage with a physiological saline
- The revival of cellular activity by vitamins, magnesium, organic silica, amino acids, and trace elements
- The reduction of the diseased calcium through mesochelation
- The use of vitamins D3 and K2 to regulate calcium transport
- The use of local anesthetics, magnesium, and anti-inflammatories to disrupt the pain cycle, providing temporary relief

---

Clinical Case: Mr. K., forty-nine years old

Knee Pain

His attending physician referred Mr. K., a civil servant, for pain in both knees, which had not responded to treatment after five years. He reported no history of trauma. His treatment consisted of anti-inflammatories, hyaluronic acid injections, and physiotherapy. Following multiple weekly treatments using the hand-syringe technique with mesochelation protocol, his knee pain improved significantly. Thanks to percutaneous hydrotomy, he no longer feels pain, and his knees are functioning optimally.

Degenerative Disc Disease

Degenerative disc disease (DDD) and disc herniation are common spine-related conditions that often occur in conjunction. A herniated disc, also known as a bulged, slipped, or ruptured disc, causes nerve pinching and severe pain, frequently in the lower back. These discs are composed of a tough outer layer called the annulus and an inner layer called the nucleus pulposis (which is 80 percent water).

In the United States, eight in ten people will experience low back pain at some point, and millions more worldwide (Freburger, 2009). Most episodes are self-limiting or resolve on their own. Low back pain increases with age, and occupational and recreational injuries are common. Obesity and smoking are also significant, modifiable risk factors. Interestingly, recent studies have shown an association between low-grade bacterial infections, such as Propionibacterium acnes, and DDD (Granville-Smith, 2022).

Most disc herniations and DDD have a mechanical and inflammatory basis that irritates the nerves, which explains the severe pain. Treatment approaches are gradual, beginning with NSAIDs and a short course of corticosteroids. Muscle relaxants may help diminish spasms and pain. Narcotics are used sparingly and only for short periods because of their addictive potential. DDD is a challenging problem, and there are no excellent treatment options. Because surgery is appropriate for only a select few, conservative treatment is recommended initially.

Intervertebral Disc Hydration

The restoration of the physiological status of the affected spinal disc segments is necessary for regeneration. Intervertebral discs have limited blood supply and rely on a process called imbibition for nutrient exchange. Imbibition is the process of water being drawn into tissue as pressure is decreased. This process explains why discs tend to rehydrate during sleep or while lying down. In fact, many studies show that after stabilization of the back through physical therapy or surgery, the intervertebral discs can undergo rehydration. While

Stopping Pain

biological attempts at disc regeneration are promising, it's important to consider other factors of DDD such as decreasing disc height, intradiscal pressure, load distribution, and motion. Studies support the theory that physiological movement and a balanced load distribution are necessary for disc regeneration (Cho, 2010; Yilmaz 2017). Given this context, regenerative injection techniques like prolotherapy, which strengthens the ligaments, may help back pain.

Many patients with DDD and pain seek percutaneous hydrotomy, which can be addressed using mesochelation or mesoperfusion techniques with hydrotomy solutions containing saline, anti-inflammatories, minerals, vitamins, amino acids, and EDTA. Most patients prefer the idea of percutaneous hydrotomy to epidural steroid injections. We have observational evidence that physiologic saline will rehydrate the discs (Guez, 2021). The contribution of magnesium, vitamins, organic silica, and especially amino acids are believed to stimulate regeneration. Finally, a vasoactive treatment is used to promote microcirculation. Our therapeutic axes are hydration, nutrition, protein synthesis, and microcirculation. We have observed few side effects, and the results are often astonishing from the first sessions. The number of treatment sessions varies between patients and depends on the severity of back pain.

There are many advantages of percutaneous hydrotomy in treating low back pain:

1. It's a nonoperative intervention that can relieve the pain through the action of local anesthetics and anti-inflammatories.
2. By injecting the tumescent state or hydrotomy cushion over the area of concern, water can diffuse to the disc region and hydrate the affected discs.

How Percutaneous Hydrotomy Treats Common Conditions

3. The water can dilute the pain mediators within the cell.
4. Minerals, such as magnesium, have a calming effect on the irritated nerves.
5. A dilute dose of corticosteroids can offer an anti-inflammatory effect and short-term relief.
6. A mesochelation or mesoperfusion protocol is used, and the number of treatments needed varies with each individual.

Clinical case: Mr. S., forty-one years old
Back Pain

My back pain was permanent despite therapy and daily painkillers following two herniated discs from motorcycle accidents. I had lost my smile because of the pain, and I was thinking of selling my motorcycle since I couldn't ride anymore without my back locking up. I came across the website www.percutaneoushydrotomy.net, which extolled the benefits of this therapy, but I didn't dare to start despite all the positive comments reported. One of my neighbors, a top cycling athlete, came by to see my tractor. After seeing me in pain as soon as I made an effort, he told me he knew of a way to alleviate my suffering. To my great astonishment, he advised me of percutaneous hydrotomy, which he knew from personal experience.

So, I went without fear to the doctor with all my examinations (X-rays, MRIs, the surgeon's report who was considering an operation). A prescription for percutaneous hydrotomy was issued. After the fifth appointment, I perceived less pain and, above all, more movement. After twelve sessions, the thing that surprised me the

> most was my wife, who, one morning, told me that she had finally rediscovered her husband, namely, my smile.
> I'm going to complete the treatments and start riding my bike again. What more can I hope for? I will get my life back. I go once a month for treatment, and I no longer take painkillers. I tinker on my motorcycle regularly. You know what, I'm alive again, and no treatment given before has allowed such a result.

Cervical Arthritis

Cervical (neck) arthritis can result from deformed cervical vertebrae (osteophytes), disc desiccation, spinal canal narrowing, and nerve compression causing pain and reduced mobility (Kuo, 2023). The primary dysfunctions are the fundamental and circulatory units, resulting in DDD. The sensation of friction between the bones results from reduced disc height. This leads to pain, neuralgia, headaches, tinnitus, and balance disorders depending on the level of cervical nerve compression. Cervical arthritis is generally treated with analgesics, anti-inflammatories, corticosteroids, and anti-seizure medications. Most patients inevitably fail on these medications, and surgery is usually recommended. The operation is not a step forward but a step backward.

The alternative in percutaneous hydrotomy is the mesochelation protocol utilizing saline, anti-inflammatories, vitamins, minerals, and EDTA to hydrate the cervical discs and restore cervical function. Mesochelation reduces diseased bone calcium, while vitamins and magnesium regenerate the damaged cartilage cells and nerves. Typically, multiple sessions are required to achieve a difference in cervical arthritis.

How Percutaneous Hydrotomy Treats Common Conditions

Rheumatoid Arthritis

Rheumatoid arthritis (RA) is a common chronic systemic inflammatory disease with primary dysfunctions in the immune and the fundamental units (Sparks, 2019). The hallmarks of RA are fatigue, symmetric joint inflammation, pain, swelling, warmth, and morning stiffness. RA affects primarily middle-aged women in their hands, wrists, feet, hips, knees, shoulders, and elbows. Cervical neck involvement is common, potentially leading to spinal instability. The prevalence of RA worldwide is approximately 1 percent of the general population (Sparks, 2019). Although the cause is unknown, the disease probably occurs in response to a pathogenic agent in a genetically predisposed host. Smoking is an environmental risk factor; other possible triggering factors include bacterial, fungal, parasitic, or viral infections.

RA is a systemic disease involving an abnormally activated immune system causing damage to the patient's own tissues. It's akin to an allergy to oneself, a phenomenon we often observe in patients who have experienced psychological and emotional trauma; for example, the death of a loved one, divorce, job loss, and aggression. One study showed that 80 percent of RA patients report depression and anxiety (Hassan, 2019).

In conventional medicine, RA is treated with immunosuppressive chemotherapy, methotrexate, NSAIDs, monoclonal antibodies, and corticosteroids. All of these treatments have undesirable long-term side effects (Sparks, 2019). Methotrexate is most commonly prescribed for RA, though it was originally designed as a chemotherapy drug (Bedoui, 2019). RA is one of the first conditions in which scientists have successfully used biological modifiers such as TNFα inhibitors (Humira™) to treat the disease. Although these

Stopping Pain

agents benefit patients with RA, cost and potential risks of toxicity limit their use.

Percutaneous hydrotomy is ideally placed to benefit RA patients. Inflammation can be reduced through the local action of water, trace minerals, anti-inflammatories, and corticosteroids. Cellular energy is optimized via the delivery of amino acids, minerals, and vitamins. The action of local anesthetics blocks the pain pathways, thus breaking the pain cycle, which is important from a psychological standpoint (Taylor, 2019).

The mesovaccination technique is sometimes employed in RA patients. When the body is immune-incompetent, it secretes chemical self-defense mediators. Think of this as a "phobia" of the skin and the mucous membranes: instead of controlling their defenses, they panic. The goal of the mesovaccination technique is to correct a failing and disorganized immunity through a staggered reeducation of its global defense system. Multiple weekly sessions are often required.

Clinical Case: Ms. A., seven years old
Rheumatoid Arthritis

Ms. A. traveled over six hundred miles with her mother, a physiotherapist, to Dr. Guez's clinic. She arrived in a wheelchair due to her juvenile polyarthritis. On examination, Ms. A. presented with edema on the right knee and ankle. Her rheumatologist prescribed her Humira™. Dr. Guez suggested a series of abdominal mesovaccination treatments to stimulate her immune defenses. A local nurse trained in percutaneous hydrotomy performed the treatments.

How Percutaneous Hydrotomy Treats Common Conditions

> Dr. Guez saw her every six months for checkups, and he observed gradual improvement. Her symptoms declined, and eventually she stopped most of her medications. By age twelve, she gave up her wheelchair, and the inflammatory flare-ups and pain disappeared. She is growing and walking normally today.

Neuropathic Pain

Neuropathic pain affects one-sixth of the US population (Campbell, 2006) and involves all five units of competency; examples are sciatic pain and herpes zoster. With neuropathic pain, nerve cells use more energy and are paralyzed and atrophied; circulation is compromised, and autoimmune reactions are common (Campbell, 2006). Protocols using percutaneous hydrotomy are aimed at all five competency areas and require a multi-specialty approach; a vasoactive treatment based on procaine, magnesium, vitamins, and vasodilators is often utilized.

> ### Clinical Case: Mrs. A., forty-seven years old
> #### Neuropathic Pain
>
> Mrs. A., a native Hawaiian, was involved in a motor vehicle accident that resulted in severe burns to her arm. Years later, she presented with severe neuropathic pain secondary to the burns. She was offered surgery to release her skin contractures and pinched nerves. She opted for percutaneous hydrotomy before going ahead with the surgery. She was treated with saline, local anesthetics,

> magnesium, procaine, amino acids, and organic silica. Initially, she experienced increased pain from her nerves "waking up." A week later, she returned for the second treatment and experienced less arm pain. Her arm pain was gone by the fourth treatment, and she no longer needed surgery. Her surgeon was perplexed, as he'd never heard of percutaneous hydrotomy.

The Skin and the Immune System

The function of the skin and immune system is essential to protect the host from an invasion of foreign organisms by distinguishing self from nonself. A well-functioning immune system protects the host from microorganisms and toxins; prevents and repels attacks by endogenous factors such as tumors; and participates in tissue repair. A normal immune response relies on a complex network of biological factors, specialized cells, tissues, and organs necessary to recognize pathogens and eliminate foreign antigens (Yasuda, 2016).

Another exciting idea is the concept of local, regional stimulation of antibodies (Yasuda, 2016). In addition, the skin contains an intricate network of resident immune cells, crucial for host defense and tissue homeostasis. In the event of an insult (injury), the skin-resident immune cells prevent infection. The deregulation of the immune response often leads to impaired healing and poor tissue restoration and function.

Allergies

Allergies cause pediatric and adult respiratory tract problems such as asthma and allergic rhinitis. These conditions result from local tissue damage and organ dysfunction in the upper and lower respiratory tracts. Allergies arise from an abnormal hypersensitive immune response to normally harmless and ubiquitous environmental allergens (Maeda, 2019). Common allergens include tree, grass, and weed pollens; others include house dust mites, cockroach antigen, mold, and animal dander. Allergic rhinitis and asthma account for significant morbidity, and atopic disorders have increased in prevalence over the past few decades.

In conventional medicine, allergen tests often yield inconsistent results (Beutner, 2023). When the nasal mucosa becomes hyperreactive to its environment, conventional medicine responds with antihistamines, corticosteroids, and antibiotics, which treat the symptoms of bacterial superinfection. But ultimately, it's our natural immune system, mitochondria, metabolic energy systems, and biological terrain that require treatment (Faas, 2020; Netea, 2020). For example, sinusitis is a dysfunction of the immune competence unit. The nasal mucosa overreacts and constantly secretes mucus. Most allergies, inflammatory diseases, and recurrent infectious diseases result from an immune disorder or incompetence called dysimmunity.

Asthma and Chronic Bronchitis

Asthma is a dysfunction of the neurological and immune system competency units and occurs when the bronchial muscles spasm, often due to hypersensitivities triggered by an allergen. Conversely, an inhaled irritant will also be naturally rejected by the body. The point to understand is that bronchial tissues no longer distinguish "friends from enemies." Chronic bronchitis results from an immune incompetence of its mucosa, leaving it unable to defend itself against allergens.

In conventional medicine, bronchodilators such as albuterol, antihistamines such as Benadryl, anti-inflammatories such as ibuprofen, and antibiotics are prescribed. Percutaneous hydrotomy focuses on the cause, that is, the immune incompetence. The body's natural defenses can be stimulated by injecting (intradermally) tiny, diluted doses of vaccines (anti-influenza, anti-Haemophilus, anti-pneumococcal). When the body regains a certain level of immune competence, the hypersensitivity and hyperreactivity of the bronchial mucosa gradually disappear, and lasting immune memory is formed. The patient becomes less fragile to their environment and can return to everyday life. Percutaneous hydrotomy aims to reduce and eliminate symptomatic treatments, and weekly sessions are typically required.

The technique of mesovaccination permits the stimulation of the immune defenses against many pathogens. Remember that the skin is one of the largest and first defenses involving our immune system. Tiny organelles called Peyer's patches are scattered throughout the skin and compose a significant part of the immune system (Yasuda, 2016; Nicolas, 2008; Combadiere, 2011). Switzerland and many other countries have used mesovaccination for many years. Many children who suffer from chronic sinusitis and ear infections can be treated by a mesovaccination protocol (Guez, 2021). It might seem logical to stimulate the immune system in the areas where the pathogens will first meet the body, in the nasal pharyngeal passages; some studies have addressed this question (Birkhoff, 2009).

Irritable Bowel Syndrome (IBS) and Colitis

Irritable bowel syndrome is a common gastrointestinal disorder affecting 10 to 15 percent of the population in Europe and the United States (Longstreth, 2006). It's associated with painful colon spasms, corresponding to immunological problems such as allergies, viruses, bacteria, and stress (Barbara, 2011). Chronic inflammation, such as rhinitis and asthma, can be secondary to these pathologies.

How Percutaneous Hydrotomy Treats Common Conditions

No pathology arrives by chance, and they all have reasons for showing their symptoms.

From a percutaneous hydrotomy perspective, IBS is a dysfunction of the neurological, immune system, and energetic competence units. Various factors can cause IBS, such as stress, surgery, long-term or repeated antibiotic therapy, immune shock to a neighboring organ, hepatitis, and infectious diseases (Barbara, 2011). The mucous membrane becomes immune-incompetent (it no longer knows how to defend itself). This imbalance leads to a reaction mode specific to all the mucous membranes; for example, inflammation, hypersecretions (phlegm), edema, pain, spasms, bloating, or bleeding.

It's necessary to emphasize the vital role of the intestinal microbiota in balancing the immune system and the triggering of autoimmune diseases (Yamamoto, 2020). The current transformation of our ecosystem leads to an imbalance of the intestinal microbiota, which is accentuated by the modern diet and pollution (heavy metals, organophosphates, and benzopyrenes) (Marynowski, 2015). The result is an irritation of the mucous membranes: sinusitis, asthma, bronchitis, recurrent cystitis, and eczema-type dermatitis.

The skin and intestines originate from the same embryonic level, which means they are mirrors of each other. This common genesis means they play a role in producing the body's immune defenses. The skin and intestines serve a fundamental role as a distribution belt between the external and internal environments, allowing the passage of trace elements, vitamins, and minerals from the diet into the bloodstream, thus making them available to the cells. The intestine also produces chemical precursors essential to hormone synthesis (serotonin, norepinephrine, dopamine, and thyroid hormone). Vitamin D is produced from cholesterol when sunlight hits our

Stopping Pain

skin; it also affects our gastrointestinal microbiome and immunity (Yamamoto, 2020).

Percutaneous hydrotomy treats IBS by supporting the immune system via mesovaccination. In our experience, mesovaccination treats intestinal dysfunction by regenerating the mucosa and is performed using a diluted polyvalent vaccine, vitamins, organic silica, and trace elements. These vaccines are obtained in Germany or Switzerland. Probiotics are also part of the treatment. Redness and edema may occur at the injection points lasting twenty-four to forty-eight hours (especially after the first session). Weekly sessions are necessary, and the long-term results remain stable and effective.

Clinical Case: Mrs. L., seventy-four years old

IBS

Mrs. L. presented to the clinic with nausea, vomiting, and recurrent abdominal pain. She was hospitalized several times for sigmoiditis (inflammation of the intestines). She was treated using mesovaccination to stimulate her immune defenses of the colon. After ten sessions her abdominal pain was gone. Over a fifteen-year follow-up, the patient had no further abdominal episodes. Her percutaneous hydrotomy treatment saved her from taking repeated antibiotics and hospitalizations, which would have led to the risk of removing part of her colon.

In chapter 8, we will explore the future of percutaneous hydrotomy, how it helps animals and athletes, and the organization and objectives of the ISPH.

Part Three
The Future—Percutaneous Hydrotomy and You

CHAPTER 8

Percutaneous Hydrotomy and the Future

Percutaneous hydrotomy has the potential to help people suffering from chronic pain. Nothing presented here is meant to be a panacea, but rather a synergy with other therapeutic strategies. While many questions remain about regenerative injection techniques, no comparative studies exist to understand which of them is most effective. The choice of technique, whether it be traditional mesotherapy or percutaneous hydrotomy or prolotherapy, depends on the patient and clinical situation. Of course, a combination of these techniques may be best for certain patients. If healthcare providers don't band together on this issue, we will all find ourselves shouting semantics at each other and regulatory institutions will take away our rights.

Healthcare providers must manage the evaluation of the techniques and effects over time. Inoculations of many mixtures of saline, minerals, anti-inflammatories, medications, herbs, and chelating agents are known, which are often based on personal conviction and sometimes based on suggestions by the pharmaceutical companies. The simplicity of these techniques is evident, and they are easily taught.

Objective proof that percutaneous hydrotomy can work for you lies in the endless testimonials found in chapter 9. Most of these patients have experienced long and arduous courses of care before coming to percutaneous hydrotomy. Our current medical system is broken. We reflexively focus on the visible symptoms of chronic pain and provide temporary relief through drugs, leaving the patient deeper in the abyss of pain. The symptoms represent only a small part of the problem. For a definitive cure, it's necessary to observe, analyze, and precisely define the root cause. In other words, you have to align the body and its function for a solution. We are firmly convinced that the future of medicine will have a closer synergy with our physiology. Using molecules familiar to our body is key.

Looking at disease through the lens of the five competencies of percutaneous hydrotomy can give us a better understanding of the root cause of a disease. Percutaneous hydrotomy helps many diseases that keep us from living a functional, complete life. Diseases causing chronic pain like arthritis and migraines can be addressed through its techniques.

The International Society of Percutaneous Hydrotomy (ISPH) organizes annual medical conferences. We continue to see notable advances, particularly in pulmonary diseases (Guez, 2022). These seemingly impossible examples help us to persevere. Our fight for percutaneous hydrotomy resembles that of David against Goliath, as the medical institutions don't help us in our research. Despite this, we are working through our actions and patient testimonials toward the day we are recognized through the mainstream medical lens. Today, the ISPH is a large group of global healthcare providers,

Percutaneous Hydrotomy and the Future

committed to the only thing that matters, which is to cure our patients, free them of chronic disease, and restore them to everyday life. It's from all these victories that we draw our strength.

Healing through the power of water, minerals, and nutrients is perhaps one of the most understudied phenomena of our age. This will likely remain due to the lack of funding for such studies. Level 1 studies, involving about one hundred people, cost approximately $1 million. However, a study on percutaneous hydrotomy in the treatment of low back pain was presented in the US at the 50th Annual Regional Anesthesiology and Acute Pain Medicine Meeting in Orlando, Florida. But let's remember these few words from Dr. Michel Pistor, the founder of mesotherapy: "Always optimistic, I believe that when the slope is favorable, like water that always flows, even if we temporarily block its way, the knowledge, too, will make its way because efficacy in innocuousness cannot stagnate for long, it will end up being universally recognized" (Sivaganam, 2010).

Many things are still possible, and the potential to improve lives is enormous if we include other animals, such as dogs and horses. Similar problems to ours already exist, such as the fight against the excessive use of pesticides and artificial fertilizers. Percutaneous hydrotomy aims to reestablish the biological terrain through regenerative medicine.

Animals and Percutaneous Hydrotomy

We are often asked if percutaneous hydrotomy can be used in animals. Veterinarians have been using it with success for many years (Saussey, 2022). French veterinarian Dr. Amelie Saussey uses percutaneous hydrotomy techniques to treat horses with musculoskeletal problems. For example, using equivalent human protocols, she treats back arthritis in many competition horses and observes an

80 percent improvement after the first treatment. She also treats herniated discs and pinched nerves. She also uses the mesostress protocols in horses with some success. Saussey is also an expert in equine acupuncture.

Dr. Veronique Lastes, also a French veterinarian, uses percutaneous hydrotomy techniques to treat dogs and cats with musculoskeletal problems. She's treated hundreds of animals, especially those cases where a contraindication for surgery exists. She presented her work at the annual conference of percutaneous hydrotomy in France and showed many cases of treating neck, back, hip, and knee problems.

Athletes and Percutaneous Hydrotomy

We are often asked if percutaneous hydrotomy is beneficial for athletes. The answer is an enthusiastic yes. We have treated many amateur and professional athletes. To date, it has been used in the following sports: MMA / UFC (see chapter 7 for the successful treatment of T.J. Dillashaw), American football (NFL), motocross, soccer, cycling, running, tennis, golf, pickleball, and baseball.

Many ask if percutaneous hydrotomy is a legal method for treating musculoskeletal injuries in sports. In the majority of sports, most regenerative injection techniques like percutaneous hydrotomy are permitted. They are referred to as WADA-approved non-doping methods (World Anti-Doping Agency, 2022). The substances and methods fall within the WADA or USADA (United States Anti-Doping Agency) guidelines. We spoke with the authorities at USADA and described the procedure in detail, and the head scientist at USADA had no issues with percutaneous hydrotomy. That said, the healthcare provider performing the procedure must stay within the guidelines of the substances used and the methods utilized (WADA, 2022). For example, corticosteroids are prohibited in some sports; in others, no more than 100 ml can be infused or injected during a six-hour period and require a therapeutic use exemption. Each sport is different, and every athlete and healthcare provider is responsible for knowing the particular rules for their sport.

The Harmonization of Pharmaceuticals

In the future, far from the current challenges (such as embarking on the race to create new complex chemical molecules), the possibilities of percutaneous hydrotomy could be expanded. This is due to the availability of new or repurposed medications. These medications will be able to extend the spectrum of our local actions on the biochemical or molecular level while avoiding any side effects.

However, we are faced with a dilemma. Many essential products in percutaneous hydrotomy, such as injectable vasodilators, certain vaccines, or EDTA, are difficult to obtain because they aren't profitable to the companies that produce them; one such example is pentoxifylline. Pharmaceutical companies have greater economic incentives to promote newer drugs for more profit, even though the existing drugs have outstanding safety records. Older drugs that are off patent are less profitable, have a high cost of regulatory compliance, and are therefore not as readily available. Fortunately, most medications used in percutaneous hydrotomy are available in several North American and European countries.

Organizations like the US Food and Drug Administration (FDA) and the European Economic Community (EEC) could harmonize the quality and safety of medicines. These are often the same laboratories that produce drugs for all countries worldwide. One current dilemma is the legislation that obliges pharmaceutical companies to produce new studies every five years for injectable products. This piece of legislation has single-handedly caused many medications to become unavailable in countries like France, yet they remain available in Italy. These studies are expensive and often do not correspond to the profitability of the drug, hence the withdrawal of many inexpensive so-called field products.

We have seen the development of increasingly expensive symptomatic treatments. This is how most injectable vasodilators have disappeared over the past twenty years; the last remaining is pentoxifylline, which has been used for over forty years in mesotherapy. The same is true for polyvalent vaccines such as Ribomunyl (used for over thirty years in chronic inflammatory diseases), which has also been withdrawn from the French market. This inconsistency in the European system means that patients in France, Germany, or Italy would have different opportunities to benefit from percutaneous hydrotomy treatments. Harmonizing pharmaceuticals is necessary to benefit the patient and the healthcare providers with the best treatments available.

The Organization and the Objectives of the International Society of Percutaneous Hydrotomy

The ISPH was created in July 2017 and includes healthcare providers from over twenty countries to improve patient care and to provide standards in the practice of percutaneous hydrotomy (Guez, 2021). A broad spectrum of medical specialties is represented: general practitioners, rheumatologists, physical medicine and rehabilitation specialists, anesthesiologists, pain specialists, otolaryngologists, nephrologists, psychiatrists, oncologists, and more. Each year, the ISPH meeting is organized in France, where ideas are exchanged and the reproducibility of our results is reinforced.

Percutaneous Hydrotomy and the Future

This structure is aimed at healthcare providers and currently pursues three primary objectives:

1. Dissemination of the technique to the public through films, interviews, and testimonials. The ISPH website, www.percutaneoushydrotomy.net, explains the technique and allows healthcare providers to understand the risks, benefits, and alternatives of percutaneous hydrotomy. Take caution: Percutaneous hydrotomy unleashes passions. Much misinformation exists on the internet from people unfamiliar with percutaneous hydrotomy or expressing unscientific opinions.
2. Recognition and scientific validation of percutaneous hydrotomy studies is underway with the United States and European Health Authorities (Ministry of Health, General Directorate of Health, High Authority for Health, National Academy of Medicine, Council of the Order of Physicians, Social Security Fund, and professional liability insurance). Communications about percutaneous hydrotomy have been presented at national and international scientific congresses (French and International Mesotherapy Societies). Memoirs from our trainee physicians were also presented as part of the interuniversity diplomas in mesotherapy; for example, Bordeaux University Hospital in 2008: Narrow Lumbar Canal and Migraines, and in 2016: Interest in Large Dilutions in Mesotherapy in the Management of Chronic Neck Pain; CHU de la Pitié-Salpêtrière in 2014 and 2017: Treatment of Knee Osteoarthritis; Claude Bernard University of Lyon in 2013: Use of EDTA in Mesotherapy Besides Osteopathic Treatment on the Cervical Osteoarthritis Spine.

3. The teaching of the percutaneous hydrotomy technique is provided by the ISPH, an approved training body. It transmits the technique to healthcare providers through theoretical courses and practical internships given in medical settings. Subsequently, continuing education, refresher courses, and research are provided throughout the year. An annual international congress brings together all healthcare providers, allowing them to exchange their ideas and experiences. These meetings are also essential for discussing the latest scientific innovations, international studies, and the global evolution of scientific knowledge beyond French borders.
- Warning: some healthcare providers are not qualified or not trained in percutaneous hydrotomy, but they still offer treatments. Inquiring on the ISPH website is imperative to connect with qualified healthcare providers.

Health Authorities and Percutaneous Hydrotomy

Institutions often don't know how to react to percutaneous hydrotomy. It's a minimally invasive and low-risk technique that allows patients to beat chronic pain and sometimes even to be cured and, therefore, to decrease or permanently stop taking medications. This technique is subversive and disruptive to the established conventional system. Economically, the percutaneous hydrotomy technique is much less profitable than other traditional allopathic techniques. Several European hospitals are employing percutaneous hydrotomy techniques to treat patients with osteoarthritis, chronic pain, postoperative pain, and high-risk cardiac conditions. Hundreds of healthcare providers are trained in percutaneous hydrotomy each year, and the technique continues to grow. Healthcare providers

Percutaneous Hydrotomy and the Future

certified to practice percutaneous hydrotomy prescribe fewer medications compared to their clinical counterparts; patients with chronic disease treated clinically are forced to endlessly buy medicines while wishing they didn't have to. This represents considerable sums of money for pharmaceutical companies and a country's healthcare system. The economic issue is essential. The financial stakes of pharmaceutical companies are significant; the turnover of drugs for 2019 alone was 60 billion euros in profit.

Changing our methods of care by abandoning medications and turning to definitive cures would be a radical metamorphosis of the Western healthcare system. It's understandable that this model, contrary to current economic models, involves complex financial and political challenges and that are costly, and time-consuming studies must be carried out. But in the meantime, a more ethical question arises: Wouldn't it be logical to promote medical freedom? Permit trusting healthcare providers, as well as the patient, to choose their mode of care. Healthcare providers practicing percutaneous hydrotomy are responsible, trained, experienced, accountable, and they comply with the ethics of their profession. They apply, with full awareness and according to current scientific knowledge, what they believe is the best for their patients.

This confrontation between economic profitability and cure shouldn't even arise. Health is not a trade; suffering is not rent. However, in a world where money dominates, priorities have changed. This was evident during the COVID-19 crisis.

A vivid example is the struggle of French physicians to gain acceptance of percutaneous hydrotomy in the mainstream medical system. The following is Dr. Guez's account of his attempts to increase the visibility of percutaneous hydrotomy techniques in France (Guez, 2021):

Stopping Pain

Fifty-four healthcare providers practicing percutaneous hydrotomy collected observations, studies, university dissertations, letters from hospital professors, exchanges with hospital university practitioners in mesotherapy, opinions from department heads in University Hospitals, scientific publications, bibliographical references, and testimonials from physicians, nurses, and patients, to present them to the National Council of the Order of Doctors (CNOM). CNOM receives 88 million euros annually from healthcare providers, organizes the election of its representatives, and gives its opinion to the state and the health authorities and is in a position to advocate for all aspects of the medical profession. However, it has done little to promote percutaneous hydrotomy. Many documents support the effectiveness of percutaneous hydrotomy have been presented to CNOM, in the face of unsolved problems in conventional medicine; however, the CNOM remains deafening silent in the face of these steps. The decisions to be taken regarding public health are urgent and are a real challenge from an economic and ecological point of view. Physicians deliver their observational studies, but it isn't their role to carry out large-scale studies. It's up to the health authorities to raise funds and select the cohorts of patients necessary for formal validations.

In 2019, Dr. Guez was received by a high-ranking individual of the French Haute Autorité de Santé (HAS), where he discussed the treatment of low back pain using percutaneous hydrotomy. At the end of the interview, Dr. Guez was told that there wasn't much that could be done, that it wasn't the role of HAS to pursue percutaneous hydrotomy, and, above all, that the pharmaceutical companies would undoubtedly oppose this concept for economic reasons.

Percutaneous Hydrotomy and the Future

Future Research in Percutaneous Hydrotomy

Water is essential to our physiology because it facilitates cellular regeneration, provides a vehicle for nutrition to cells, and is a vector for transmitting energy. All cells emit electromagnetic waves, which differ depending on the cell's water content. If the cell is diseased, cancerous, infected by a pathogen, or has DNA damage, the emission of these waves is no longer the same. The ability to detect these cellular wave emissions by a receiving device would be an advancement in medicine. Modifying these different electromagnetic waves with water could restore a cell's healthy state. For example, it has been shown that electromagnetic induction can block action potentials to decrease nervous transmission in sensory and in motor neurons, producing anesthesia (Ye, 2022; Hashemi, 2019). Avenues like this need exploring, and future healthcare providers will be interested in choosing the physical route rather than a chemical one.

We've seen throughout this book that percutaneous hydrotomy aims to heal, repair, and regenerate human tissue using the power of water. By using molecular physics, water can also destroy cells. Dr. Michel Pistor and others had thought of developing a controlled delivery of hypertonic water to kill diseased cells in cancers, metastases, nodules, lymphomas, and small tumors. The idea was to use longer needles that could reach deep tumors. Interventional ultrasound and CT didn't yet exist; therefore, this idea wasn't workable, but today it can become a reality. One could create extracorporeal infusions connected to long needles (5, 10, 15 cm), all guided by ultrasound or CT to reach deep tumors (e.g., hepatic). The water used would no longer be isotonic but hypertonic or hypotonic—that is, the osmotic pressure of the water would differ from that contained in the failing cell. We could thus disrupt the membranes of cancerous cells. With a precise concentration gradient, we can generate the programmed disintegration of the cell, and computers would control this destruction to respect the precise area concerned (Kaplan, 1988).

A Final Word about Percutaneous Hydrotomy

We are often asked what percutaneous hydrotomy is and where it fits into the treatment spectrum. First and foremost, it is not a panacea. It's just one of the many regenerative injection techniques that exist today. The best way to think about it is regarding the numerous options you have with certain maladies. For example, if you have appendicitis, a life-threatening infection of the appendix, you don't have many options. In most cases appendicitis must be treated with antibiotics and often surgically removed to prevent further infection. But when you have a chronic disease like knee arthritis, there are many treatment options. Think of the treatment options for knee pain as a buffet. In a sense, you can choose what to put on your plate. It may be that you start with taking an NSAID for the osteoarthritis and getting an X-ray. Then later, a regenerative injection technique like platelet-rich plasma (PRP) is another treatment that can help. In some cases, it will treat the knee pain and that is all you will need to do. In others, it is a bridge to increase your function until it is time to have a knee replacement.

In the business of medicine, it costs millions to bring a medical product to market and get it approved by an organization like the FDA. Since no pharmaceutical or medical company stands to make billions of dollars from regenerative medical procedures like percutaneous hydrotomy, prolotherapy, or perineural injections, it is unlikely there will ever be funded trials or sponsored research in this area. It should also be remembered that it takes about $1 million

Percutaneous Hydrotomy and the Future

to do a level 1 research study in musculoskeletal diseases. One of the few ways for these techniques to become an accepted method for treatment is through books, the press, and self-funded research. Treatments such as percutaneous hydrotomy will always lie outside mainstream medicine's "standard of care." At this time, only PRP and stem cell therapies are profitable for medical companies and are thus highly promoted.

What evidence is there that there's any validity to percutaneous hydrotomy? Many ask, where are the studies? It is true, few studies exist in the literature; the ones published are in French (Guez, 2021). However, it's important to realize that percutaneous hydrotomy is the culmination of several techniques that have all been thoroughly studied and found to be safe and effective. Several studies exist about the efficacy of regenerative injection therapies. For example, there are hundreds of studies on mesotherapy, tumescent therapy, hypodermoclysis, and prolotherapy. We can attest to the benefits of percutaneous hydrotomy from our experiences of hundreds of thousands of procedures performed on several thousand patients. Apart from anecdotal evidence, our data comes from the literature, attending conferences, courses, and the numerous healthcare practitioners who practice the technique in over twenty-five countries. The data we have is of course not perfect, and neither is any data from orthopedic or pain medicine literature, for example. We often review and change our practice of medicine according to newer literature and patient outcomes. At the end of the day, we make the best treatment choices for our patients to achieve the best outcome. Cutting-edge doctors still rely on case reports and case series as a way to find new techniques.

Finally, it is estimated that over one million percutaneous hydrotomy procedures have been safely performed by trained healthcare providers worldwide. Our hope is that interested healthcare providers will learn this simple and effective regenerative injection technique and perform research and publish their findings. We are confident that percutaneous hydrotomy will help patients and provide another option for those suffering from chronic pain.

Hopefully you can appreciate some of the intricacies of delivering percutaneous hydrotomy to the public, alternative patient populations such as animals and athletes, and the roadblocks that alternative and complementary medicine faces against the colossal pharmaceutical companies. Yet, the truth always burns in the flame. It burns off the dead wood. And people don't like having the dead wood burned off. In the next chapter, you will read about the countless patient testimonials that are truly at the core of percutaneous hydrotomy. Percutaneous hydrotomy could also become a new experimental method for studying drug interactions and skin-based mechanisms. Those who practice this technique by correctly selecting the patients to be treated, aiming to reduce localized pain and the doses of systemic drugs, will discover its therapeutic value. Healthcare providers should take advantage of this technique to facilitate the treatment path of many patients. Of course, many scientific questions remain, but one must be open to the goal, expand upon the research, and not discard the hypothesis: if a medicine works, but we do not know why, we should not refuse it.

CHAPTER 9

Giving the Floor to the Patients: Testimonials

This is perhaps the most powerful chapter in this book, because the examples herein are from actual patients, with real results. The ISPH organized a testimonial session over three months with the help of our healthcare providers trained in percutaneous hydrotomy. The patients were asked to describe their course of treatment in conventional medicine and then their treatment in percutaneous hydrotomy. We've received thousands of testimonials relating to various chronic diseases. Only a small sample of these testimonials are presented; the patients' names are kept anonymous to preserve medical privacy. Hopefully, these results can give you the motivation to consider percutaneous hydrotomy for yourself. Many of these patients are nurses, physicians, firemen, police officers, and office workers.

Note: Many of these testimonials are translated from French.

Stopping Pain

Migraines

Madame J., forty-eight years old, migraines, mesochelation
I've been suffering from migraines for over thirty years. In 2015, I felt an increase in the attacks. I started by treating the attacks with triptans, a drug prescribed by the general practitioner. A neurologist also followed me for nine months. This treatment reduced the intensity of the seizures. After this treatment, I continued with the triptans in case of crisis. In 2017, I started having constant pain in the left side of my head, and even triptans and anti-inflammatories didn't work. I started doing physiotherapy, osteopathy, and chiropractic sessions without much result. I had a cervical nerve decompression operation in December 2017. Three months later, I had fewer migraines, but the left-sided pain continued. I was diagnosed with Arnold's neuralgia and cervical spondylosis at that time. I continued with the physiotherapy and chiropractic sessions, which provided some relief. I learned about percutaneous hydrotomy on social media from a man being treated for Arnold's neuralgia. After seeing a doctor, I started the infusion sessions, twelve total, once a week. At the start of the sessions, I had an increased number of attacks, but positive results came from the seventh and eighth sessions. Today, I have attacks from time to time, but nothing bad. For me, it's simply a new life.

Miss M., twenty-seven years old, migraines, mesochelation
I have suffered for almost three years from Arnold's neuralgia and trigeminal neuralgia, an extremely painful pathology. Before getting to know Mr. M. and percutaneous hydrotomy, I met around fifty caregivers (neurologist, neurosurgeon, pain center doctor, osteopath, and chiropractor, to name a few). I was on morphine and

Giving the Floor to the Patients: Testimonials

Laroxyl, an antidepressant. Unable to get out of bed many days, the illness and the pain led me straight into a deep depression. I crossed paths with Mr. M. and started percutaneous hydrotomy treatments. After about ten sessions, gradually, my pain subsided, and I regained a real quality of life. I resumed swimming, my studies, and making plans. For me, percutaneous hydrotomy is my miracle solution. Since I started the treatments, I stopped the morphine and the antidepressants and decreased the Laroxyl, from twenty-five to five drops. With all my heart, I hope my testimony will allow percutaneous hydrotomy to be recognized by Social Security and reimbursed because everyone deserves to be treated as they should be!

Madame F., seventy-four years old, migraines and Arnold's neuralgia, mesochelation
For two years, I've suffered from Arnold's neuralgia, which gives me terrible headaches at the base and sides of my skull. After physiotherapy, osteotherapy, acupuncture, and analgesic medications, I had no results. One day, a friend undergoing percutaneous hydrotomy recommended this treatment to me after it gave her some relief. So, I started the treatments in December 2018, and I felt a marked improvement from the third injection. I finished the injections (ten times in three months), and I'm delighted. I have regained sleep and the pleasure of moving, of going out. In a word, I'm alive again, thanks to percutaneous hydrotomy.

Madame S., fifty-eight years old, migraines and neck pain, mesochelation
From September 2017 to May 2018, I had numerous sick leaves due to cervical neck pain and, ultimately, Arnold's neuralgia. I had unbearable pain, visual disturbances, loss of balance, and the

pain intensified with effort. Amid a crisis, it was impossible to remain standing, with only one solution—total rest. No treatment could give me lasting relief: anti-inflammatories, analgesics, cortisone infiltrations, numerous physiotherapy sessions, and acupuncture. In March 2018, I started the percutaneous hydrotomy treatments. By the fourth session, I experienced a marked improvement, and on the sixth, no more pain. I underwent about twenty injections in total. I returned to work in June. In August, I had sciatica. I started the infusions, and the pain disappeared little by little after about ten injections. At the end of all this, I went back to work, followed the course of my life, and resumed sports and hiking.

Shoulder Pain

Madame L., sixty years old, shoulder pain, mesochelation
In February 2015, I experienced severe left shoulder pain and severely reduced range of motion. I consulted my doctor and was diagnosed with shoulder tendinitis and given an injection of cortisone and oral anti-inflammatories. An X-ray showed calcifying tendinitis of the supraspinatus, approximately 8 mm. After a month and a half, the intense pain returned. I consulted my doctor again, and he recommended physiotherapy sessions while continuing with anti-inflammatories and painkillers. After twenty sessions of physiotherapy and the medications, the pain was a little less but omnipresent. Tolerating my pain, I resigned to living with it, but after several months, the pain became worse with more throbbing. So again, I consulted my doctor, and he gave me another injection and a prescription for anti-inflammatories. It relieved the pain a little at the moment, but not over time. In September 2017, I could no longer sleep and could no longer place my arm in a position to avoid

Giving the Floor to the Patients: Testimonials

pain. Yet again, I consulted my doctor, and he said, "We are going to do an MRI for an operation since the other treatments have not worked." In September 2017, the results of the MRI showed calcification of the infra and supraspinatus tendons measuring 14 mm. Not only did the treatments fail to work, but the calcifications worsened. I hesitated to have the operation because someone I know had it, and even several months later was not doing well. So, I gave myself some time to reflect. In January 2018, the pain became too much, and I searched for alternatives to the operation. I researched on the internet and came across some testimonials of percutaneous hydrotomy. After asking a few questions, I made an appointment with the practitioners. I was prescribed weekly treatments, and my first session was in March 2018. I felt relief after the second session because I finally got back to sleep, and the pain was less present at night. I regained the mobility of my shoulder. After the following sessions, I felt, from week to week, a decrease in my pain. So, I did my twelve sessions. I went to see my surgeon in June 2018. I explained to him that I had done twelve percutaneous hydrotomy sessions, and he listened to me, but didn't comment. He examined my shoulder and did all the necessary movements to check the mobility, and he said, "Good, well, I see that you have regained great mobility, so for me, no operation. I will send the report to your attending physician." I can live again today because I can use my arm without concern or pain. I also had a popliteal cyst treated by hydrotomy, and again, what a relief. Looking back, I wonder why our healthcare providers don't offer this treatment. It would cost Social Security much less than an operation, hospitalization, and rehabilitation.

Today, I'm no longer in pain, and I forgot to mention that I do a lot of dancing. I went to the Avoriaz festival this summer

Stopping Pain

for over a week with twenty-one hours of lessons in addition to all the evenings. My arms and shoulders worked great and were pain free. Today, I would like to say a big thank you to the whole team who practices percutaneous hydrotomy and who are fighting to ensure that this practice is recognized, because it's worth it for the patients.

Madame D., seventy-two years old, neck and shoulder pain, mesochelation
I developed left shoulder pain in January 2017. An ultrasound showed calcifications in my tendons, acromioclavicular bursitis, biceps tendinopathy, and tears in my rotator cuff. I then developed right shoulder pain in April 2018. Using my arm for simple acts like peeling vegetables became very difficult. After two months of percutaneous hydrotomy treatments, I can use my arm and walk again. I've rediscovered well-being and ease in normal daily movements. I've reduced my tramadol tablets (one tablet instead of six per day). How can you not believe in this medicine? Thank you to percutaneous hydrotomy for allowing me to resume a more pleasant life.

Mr. R., twenty-four years old, rotator cuff injury
I am a professional motorcycle racer, and I came to see Dr. Edwards after injuring my shoulder. I could not move my arm, and it was pinned to my side and painful, especially at night. The MRI showed that I had multiple rotator cuff injuries, but nothing was completely torn. I was desperate for help since my season started in six weeks and I did not want to undergo surgery. A fellow racer told me about Dr. Edwards, so I went to his clinic. He suggested treatment of percutaneous hydrotomy combined with PRP injections into my shoulder for four weeks. After the initial session, I experienced significant

relief, which allowed me to increase my shoulder rehabilitation. Finally, by week four I regained nearly full shoulder mobility, and I could ride again. I started my season on time, and although not perfect, my shoulder's condition exceeded my expectations thanks to Dr. Edwards's treatment.

Neck and Back Pain

Madame H., fifty-six years old, back pain, mesoperfusion
My back pain began in February 2017, which put me down for many months. I underwent many treatments which completely wiped me out, but didn't take away the pain. I could no longer do my normal job as a childcare assistant in the maternity ward on the night shift. I couldn't dance or play sports (usually four to five hours a week). I had to start taking antidepressants. I met with two neurosurgeons. One recommended surgery without certainty of results, and the other did not recommend surgery. I decided against surgery. Thanks to a friend, I got in touch with F. and B., who introduced me to percutaneous hydrotomy. My saviors! I had twenty-four sessions of mesoperfusion hydrotomy at the rate of one session per week for the first few months, as prescribed by Dr. Z. It was only around the end of the fifteenth session that I could resume some activities. I remained sick for nine months. In November 2018, I resumed my part-time therapeutic activity for five months and eventually resumed full-time. Today, I do Pilates twice weekly; I have resumed dance classes and even go out dancing. I'm living again! To date, I do maintenance treatments every three weeks. Since the beginning, I have been in treatment with a physiotherapist twice weekly. I also consulted my osteopath and a naturopath, who are familiar with percutaneous hydrotomy. I have a follow-up with the latter with a change of diet and food supplements. I can't thank B. and

Stopping Pain

F. enough for their listening, patience, encouragement, care, and professionalism. They were a great support. After these treatments, I have had a real positive evolution, that is to say, much less paresthesia and no more pain.

Madame S., fifty-one years old, neck and back pain, mesoperfusion
I was on my daily bike ride when a drunk driver ran me over in May 2015. He was also on antidepressants and didn't see me. In my misfortune, I found myself flying through the air and sustained vertebral fractures at L1 and L3. After being hospitalized for three weeks, I returned home. I found it impossible to sit or stand for more than five minutes. I was left to deal with lower neck and back and pain as well as paresthesia in my neck upon leaving the hospital. I was taking many medications, but the pains were still present. The nights were endless. I could only sleep on my back, with pain waking me up. I quickly returned to a state of fatigue that I couldn't overcome. Despite all that, I kept my spirits up and told myself that it was a bad time to die and that it would pass. At the end of the fifth month, I started driving to the physiotherapist, who was five kilometers from my house. I wanted to regain some independence. And then I realized it wouldn't be as easy as I thought. I did not have autonomy and needed a belt to support my back. I was stiff as a post, had trouble seeing, and didn't feel safe. What created the most anxiety and fear was that I no longer recognized myself. And I was talking to myself: "It's going to be fine. You've always been driven. You can do it."

Medically, the vertebrae were healing, and the equipment was in place. The surgeon had done an excellent job, but the braces created stiffness in my back and neck and considerable loss of mobility, and daily pain that impacted my life. It was impossible to go shopping,

Giving the Floor to the Patients: Testimonials

do household chores, cook, wash, and dress. Depending on the time, I still needed help. The only place where I felt good was in the water, so I did water therapy to regain mobility. Following low back pain, an MRI was prescribed for me: degenerative disc disease from L5 to S1. A cervical neck MRI showed that I had a moderate inversion of the curvature on C5 / C6 and C6 / C7, as well as the beginnings of moderate progressive disc disease. It was in February 2017 that the surgeon told me that the braces were finally going to be removed. My vertebrae were healed. The braces handicapped me, but he told me I would regain mobility and reduce my pain. The surgeon told me that the operation is straightforward. Under general anesthesia, he would reopen the four scars, remove the equipment, and in the evening, I would go home. Well, that was in theory because, in reality, I suffered martyrdom for two months. I had returned to the starting point. I could no longer wash, dress, cook, or do any household chores; I couldn't even go out to walk. It was a descent into hell for me between February 2017 and November 2018. After three and a half years of working with physiotherapists, osteopaths, acupuncturists, swimming pools, doctors, surgeons, and psychologists, the pains were still ruining my life. It was impossible to find a comfortable position to fall asleep at bedtime. I woke up 3 times a night due to back pain, or neck pain, having to get up to walk. Everything scared me, and I only felt safe at home. To keep from going crazy, I took medication that relieved me for a while and put me in a trance. One morning in February 2018, I said: "There, that's enough! You have to do something. It can't go on like this." I went to my doctor, who told me I had depression, an attack of anxiety and fear. It's the aftermath of the accident. He made me understand that I first had to accept the disability and to find the right balance of what I could do. The pains, unfortunately, will be for life. And that the only way to

Stopping Pain

stop them was through sports and strengthening myself. He put me on medications to manage my anxieties and my fears. Throughout my journey, no one gave me a solution to my pain, apart from medication that put me in a daze and only relieved me for a short time. In October 2018, I accompanied my mom to her appointment, and since Mrs. H. treats me with homeopathy, I thought, why not give it a try? I remember my first appointment. Mrs. H. looked at my X-rays and said, "You must be in pain." I told her that's why I was there. After explaining what I had been going through daily for three and a half years, she offered me percutaneous hydrotomy treatments. And there, I said to myself, finally, a medicine that offers me a more natural treatment. I didn't hesitate for a second. We started by treating my back with an infusion called "the octopus," consisting of eighteen needles with 500 ml of solution. The results were fast. From the second week, I felt a sense of well-being that I had forgotten. I did ten sessions, and today I no longer have the pain I had every day. Sitting and standing static is no longer a problem. Taking the car to get around no longer scares me. I have regained my mobility and resumed my activities. And above all, I feel serene, as if I were living again and with no more medications. What happiness.

At the cervical level, hydrotomy is done by hand syringe, and a needle is injected into several points. The results are spectacular, a clear improvement from the second week. By the fifth week, there was no more radiation or pain in my head. My neck is much more flexible, and I have regained serenity. I get up in the morning rested and can think. Incredible! Also, I no longer take any medication. If you had told me, I wouldn't believe it. But this is me who experienced it. I continue my sessions at the cervical level, but already my life has completely changed.

Giving the Floor to the Patients: Testimonials

Mr. G., forty-five years old, neck pain, mesochelation
I've had cervical neuralgia-type pain for more than fifteen months (VAS 9/10 at night). I had to take Oxycodone 10 mg for more than six months. The MRI shows four herniated discs, C2–C3, C3–C4, C4–C5, and C6–C7, with a narrow cervical canal C6–C7 showing signs of spinal cord injury. After four sessions of percutaneous hydrotomy, I discontinued all analgesics. After one year, I had no more pain or paresthesia, and I recovered strength in my right hand. The MRI of February 2019 shows the disappearance of the narrow cervical canal and the absence of pain. Percutaneous hydrotomy avoided surgery in my case.

Mr. C., forty-nine years old, back pain, mesoperfusion
I'm a sports educator, athlete, and a competitor. I consulted my general practitioner after having lower back pain, which handicapped my left leg with intense pain when sitting and lying down. He prescribed me anti-inflammatories for fifteen days; however, the pain persisted. I went back to see my doctor, who again prescribed me anti-inflammatories with physiotherapy and osteopathy sessions, but the pain persisted despite these sessions. After my insistence, a CT scan of the lumbar spine revealed the presence of L5–S1 discopathy with a herniated left posterolateral disc and left foraminal, causing sciatica for about three months. The pain was unbearable, so I underwent an infiltration of corticosteroids under fluoroscopy, but the pain persisted, and surgery was recommended to me to treat this herniated disc. I refused the operation.

    I have worked with a naturopathic doctor for several years and am convinced about the benefits of oral hypertonic Quinton water

Stopping Pain

treatments. My naturopath told me about physiologic saline injections to treat herniated discs and other pathologies.

After researching a qualified medical practitioner, I made an appointment with Dr. H. to establish a protocol to treat my herniated disc with percutaneous hydrotomy. He directed me to Mrs. M., a nurse trained in hydrotomy. The biweekly treatments lasted one hour, and the nurse placed twelve needles in the lumbar region as specified by Dr. H. After only five sessions of percutaneous hydrotomy, I felt a clear improvement, despite the intensive continuation of my training and preparation for my competitions.

The protocol of twelve sessions will be enough to free me from this pain. How could I suffer for months with medication without any positive effect and an operation proposal when the solution was in front of me? No more permanent moral exhaustion, no more pain with every movement day and night, no more clenching your teeth in pain while driving. I wake up rested. Percutaneous hydrotomy injections cured me of my herniated disc, and I continue to show permanent healing today. I talk about it to everyone who has not found a solution to their problems with medication. The idea of being unable to treat themselves and continue living normally was unbearable for me. This can cure specific pathologies without side effects, without making people addicted to drugs with disastrous effects for the body, before letting them sink into a depression engendered by permanent pain. Everyone must be free to choose what is best for their body. If I had listened to the pressure of the doctors, I would have had the operation, and perhaps the operation would have been a success, as is often the case for many people. But I'm happy to have been able to avoid it, and if one day the pain returns, it's certain that percutaneous hydrotomy will cure me.

Giving the Floor to the Patients: Testimonials

Mr. P., fifty-seven years old, back pain, mesoperfusion
I am a healthcare practitioner who has practiced osteopathy and physiotherapy for over thirty years. I sustained an L5–S1 disc herniation in 1989 following an effort to prevent a patient from falling. I didn't have an operation, but I did develop osteoarthritis. More recently, I herniated a disc at C5–C6 and found out that I had cervical osteoarthritis. I have significant cervical pain affecting my right arm. I underwent percutaneous hydrotomy treatments for eighteen months: ten lumbar infusions and ten hand-syringe injections in my lumbar area. I also had ten injections in my cervical area. The results: lumbar stiffness regressed, no more pain, and a clear improvement at the cervical level. I regularly refer patients to percutaneous hydrotomy practitioners and I've received only good or excellent feedback.

Madame B., sixty-seven years old, back pain, mesoperfusion
Ten years ago, I had surgery for a herniated disc. In 2017, suffering from a second herniated disc with nerve damage, I was bedridden for two months and lost a tremendous amount of weight. I no longer slept, no longer ate, and the pain was present despite taking a battery of drugs. Ultimately, the two surgeons I consulted wanted to operate on me. I found this percutaneous hydrotomy method by Dr. Guez on the internet; I contacted Mr. M., who gave me information about the procedure. From the first sessions, I regained the feeling of my skin on the tibia, which was like touching cardboard. I continued the hydrotomy sessions during November, December 2017, January, February, March, April, May, and June 2018, at one session per week, then one session every two weeks. I walk normally, and I live normally. All my scans, reports, and other examinations support my testimony of healing.

Stopping Pain

Mr. T., thirty-four years old, back pain, mesoperfusion
I, Mr. T., police officer, have received percutaneous hydrotomy care. Without this care, I would never have been able to recover so quickly from my cervical herniated disc, which had made me suffer for six months. I saw a neurosurgeon, and he was planning to operate on me. To date, I no longer suffer, and I've had no relapse for my hernia so that I could resume my various physical activities (boxing, bodybuilding) without any discomfort.

Hand Pain

Madame M., fifty-five years old, hand pain, mesochelation
I've suffered from digital osteoarthritis localized on the two index fingers and the little finger of the right hand for about six years. This caused deformities in the joints and resulted in attacks of pain, sometimes intense enough to bother me in certain circumstances:

- my professional practice (I write a lot by hand or on a computer)
- when I was driving
- during sleep

When I consulted my doctor, he admitted that he was helpless in facing this irreversible problem. He prescribed me painkillers and anti-inflammatories to take with each attack. The problem, therefore, remained without a satisfactory solution, especially since I did not want to abuse anti-inflammatories. Last year, I heard about percutaneous hydrotomy and saw Dr. N., who prescribed me twelve sessions. Madame J., a nurse, took care of me afterward. The treatments started in October 2018 and stopped at the beginning of

Giving the Floor to the Patients: Testimonials

January 2019. Even though my finger joints remain deformed, they don't cause pain. It's a relief for me, and will likely work for at least another ten years, not to mention the daily tasks. I recommend this technique to those around me without any reservations.

Knee Pain

Madame P., sixty-four years old, knee pain, mesochelation
I've suffered from knee pain for thirty years, following the dislocation of my kneecaps that were poorly treated from the start. It resulted in patellar misalignment, stiffness in the knee joint, progressively significant cartilage wear extending to both knees, and the gradual onset of osteoarthritis. Over the years, the pain set in, and my quality of life deteriorated: pain going up and down stairs, total inability to squat and get up from the ground, pain during physical activities such as cycling and walking, to the point of having to stop all the activities. I tried to remedy this state of affairs by taking painkillers, the effectiveness of which gradually diminished. Four years ago, I tried hyaluronic acid injections, which were ineffective as far as I was concerned. My doctor then prescribed physiotherapy sessions, which showed the damage but didn't bring relief. In October 2017, a neighbor familiar with this process encouraged me to attend a conference by Dr. Bernard Guez on percutaneous hydrotomy. I was impressed with the explanation and the results shown at the conference. I decided to try it and benefited from a series of twelve sessions per knee between May 2018 and February 2019. After a few sessions, I felt an improvement in the pain and, little by little, my joints became more flexible, the movements were carried out with more fluidity and amplitude. My daily life has improved, and I've started to evolve again in an appreciable comfort of life. Feeling more

Stopping Pain

confident and solid on my legs, I resumed walking and cycling on uneven or slightly uneven terrain. Since the beginning of percutaneous hydrotomy care, I have not taken painkillers. I rediscovered pleasure in physical activity, and my overall health improved. To consolidate the care, on the advice of the nurse and the doctor, I've just started the second series of twelve sessions in total, spread over time. The positive effects continue to develop. In conclusion, I can now objectively see the benefits of hydrotomy on my joint problems, related to osteoarthritis in particular. A perspective other than a total joint replacement is now open to me. I hope that percutaneous hydrotomy will continue to be financially accessible to patients who see a significant improvement in their health thanks to this approach.

Mr. L., sixty-eight years old, knee pain, mesochelation
I love golf, and I played about 130 courses per year, walking nearly ten kilometers each time. Following various life accidents in 2005, I had severe knee pain. X-rays of my knees in 2010 and 2014 showed that I had very advanced osteoarthritis and was advised to have surgery. The rheumatologist injected my knees with hyaluronic acid twice per year, for four years, with results difficult to comprehend. In 2014, an MRI of my left knee showed that my knee was bone-on-bone, and the radiologist was surprised that I could even walk! Walking was causing significant pain, so I considered stopping golf. In January 2017, I met Dr. Guez, who advised that I try percutaneous hydrotomy. After the first injections, I must say that the results were almost immediate. I persisted, and after several injections, the pain was practically gone. In September 2016, I injured my left shoulder rotator cuff. I refused the operation. I

Giving the Floor to the Patients: Testimonials

had percutaneous hydrotomy injections in May 2017, with excellent results. Today, I play about 150 golf courses a year. I always have slight pain at the end of the course. I'm delighted with the results and think the health authorities should be interested in this technique.

Madame R., sixty-eight years old, knee pain, mesochelation
After forty years of working on my knees doing indoor restoration, my knees had suffered enormously. Ten years ago, I underwent an operation for each knee to remove the pieces of cartilage that had deteriorated and were causing me pain. But I remained fragile and experienced pain while walking or playing sports. From the first session of percutaneous hydrotomy, I felt a new comfort. I'm in the third session, and I have no more pain. The result has been miraculous and I'm delighted because the result is unexpected and natural.

Foot / Ankle Pain
Madame B., fifty-one years old, foot pain, mesochelation
I've been suffering for nearly two years from acute pain in my left foot, seriously handicapping me. These pains are located in the front of my foot, at the level of the metatarsus. I underwent many examinations to define the causes, which seem to be due to osteoarthritis. Nothing has been able to relieve my pain so far. Six weeks ago, I started percutaneous hydrotomy injections and felt an improvement from the first session. Indeed, I have had six injections so far, and I can finally walk normally (I was limping and couldn't stand for long periods). I have regained a normal personal and professional life.

Stopping Pain

Mr. J., twenty-one years old, chronic ankle and knee pain
Mr. J., a young college soccer player, struggled with chronic ankle and knee pain due to multiple soccer-related injuries, including a torn knee meniscus, ankle injury, ACL rupture, and medial collateral ligament tears. After a year of extensive rehabilitation, Mr. J.'s return was marred by persistent knee stiffness and pain. Despite efforts to play through the discomfort, the pain only intensified, and he considered giving up the sport he loved. Given the demanding schedule of college soccer, Mr. J. knew he had to find a solution for his injuries. He'd exhausted conventional treatments, including anti-inflammatories, physical therapy, stretching, and icing. Surgery was offered, but it would end his season. A friend introduced Mr. J. to Dr. Edwards, who suggested that Mr. J. try percutaneous hydrotomy. Intrigued and desperate for a solution, Mr. J., supported by his parents, underwent the treatment. Mr. J.'s ankle and knee were injected with a solution containing anti-inflammatories, minerals, magnesium, amino acids, local anesthetics, and a trace amount of steroids. Mr. J. tested his knee and ankle through running and other physical activities. To his relief, he experienced significant improvement. He did two additional treatments. Mr. J. shared his experience in a testimonial, noting how the treatment had allowed him to return to soccer full-time and prepare for the upcoming season. He now harbors hope of playing professionally.

Mr. J.'s Testimonial

"My experience with Dr. Edwards is one that I am forever thankful for. I went through a series of sports injuries involving tears to my ACL, lateral and medial meniscus, and my medial collateral ligament. I was out of sports and doing rehab for over a year. When I

Giving the Floor to the Patients: Testimonials

was getting closer to returning to sports, I felt confident and happy with my progress, but then I started to feel an overwhelming amount of stiffness and pain in my knee while performing in my sport. As time went on, I would push through the pain in hopes that it would go away, but it only progressed. Even more, my condition put me in a frustrated and confused state of mind. I never thought in my life that I would start to lose my passion for soccer, a sport to which I've dedicated my whole life. But with the pain I was playing through on a daily basis, I didn't see a future continuing to play like this unless I found a solution to the pain. When I got introduced to Dr. Edwards, I told him what I was experiencing and how I functioned daily. He proposed to me the percutaneous hydrotomy treatment that he could inject around my kneecap and the potential benefits it had to offer. After further learning about the shot and its benefits, I immediately agreed to the process. I knew my good friend had benefited greatly from percutaneous hydrotomy, so I knew it would be safe to try. After my first round of percutaneous hydrotomy, I gave my knee a day or two to settle in before putting it through physical activity to test it. I started running and doing my normal activities. I immediately noticed the difference, and there was no painful reaction to my movements. I was in shock and overcome with joy, and my smile while playing the sport I loved returned. I have full confidence in my actions. It is all thanks to Dr. Edwards and the amazing treatment he has to offer. I highly suggest that anyone going through any chronic pain or overwhelming stiffness that won't go away check out Dr. Edwards. You will be amazed at how well percutaneous hydrotomy works."

Madame B., ankle pain, mesochelation
About three years ago, I had great difficulty walking for more than a few minutes due to severe pain in my left ankle, which swelled

Stopping Pain

quickly, especially in hot weather, apparently related to osteoarthritis. For a very long time, I've had a fragility of the ankle tendons, which made me regularly twist my ankle with a lateral tilting of my foot, a phenomenon that has become more frequent. An orthopedic surgeon recommended a series of physiotherapy massages. I learned about Dr. Guez from one of his patients, who was very satisfied with her results. After much hesitation and doubt, I finally decided to try it myself. At the rate of one session per week in the beginning, then every three to four weeks, the condition of my ankle gradually and considerably improved, allowing me to regain function and decrease my pain. I was able to walk again. I'm delighted with this result which has changed my life, and currently, one session every six weeks allows me to maintain it perfectly. For my part, I can, therefore, only speak of percutaneous hydrotomy in the most positive way.

Mr. E., fifty-four years old, ankle injury, mesochelation
While playing tennis, I rolled my left ankle, leading to immediate pain and swelling. Initially, I thought it was broken due to the intense pain and inability to bear weight. I took painkillers, rested, and underwent hyperbaric oxygen therapy (HBOT), expecting surgery.

Surprisingly, the X-rays the next day showed no fracture to my amazement and the orthopedic surgeon concluded that I had strained or partially torn the anterior fibular ligament. I was offered percutaneous hydrotomy to accelerate the healing which included a solution of saline, lidocaine, magnesium, amino acids, procaine, pentoxifylline, B vitamins, trace minerals, and a tiny dose of anti-inflammatories. I followed the percutaneous hydrotomy session with HBOT. Within two weeks I resumed activity.

Giving the Floor to the Patients: Testimonials

I again repeated the percutaneous hydrotomy and two hours of HBOT. By this time, the swelling and bruising had gone down considerably. I felt stable standing on my ankle and decided I might try to gently hit some tennis balls the next day. At three weeks post-injury I repeated the percutaneous hydrotomy and HBOT and I started hitting tennis balls with no side-to-side movement. My ankle felt stable, considering the severity of the sprain. It was apparent all the rehab and interventions I had done thus far had paid off for my ankle injury. Four weeks post-injury I hit for an hour with my tennis coach. I decided to start playing tennis again and signed up for a tournament I had wanted to play in but without expectations. I played three clay matches without any problems. Nearly six weeks after injuring my ankle, I played in a tennis tournament, and again, my ankle felt fine. My ankle was completely healed. I was discussing my ankle injury with some other tennis players, and they couldn't believe that my ankle had recovered in only six weeks at my age of fifty-four years old. I had a total of four percutaneous hydrotomy treatments, and numerous hours of HBOT.

Eczema, Bronchitis, and Allergies

Madame G., thirty years old, eczema, mesovaccination
Two years ago, I started to suffer from eczema attacks. I don't know what triggered these crises, but they have become regular. Last September, I suffered a crisis with infected pimples all over my body, extreme itching day and night (I got up three times a night on average to reapply the creams), but also a constantly red and puffy face. The itching became so violent that I was left with raw skin that could no longer heal, so I put compresses fixed with adhesive plaster. Also, I work at a public job, so I was all

Stopping Pain

the more embarrassed, which affected my morale. I felt terrible about myself.

I went to the Saint-Louis Hospital in Paris, renowned in dermatology. A dermatologist physician prescribed me corticosteroid creams and antihistamines, which I took twice daily. An intern at the consultation remarked, "It's your disease. You have to get used to it!" This little sentence was tough to hear because I could not envision my life under these conditions. I also tried essential oils, but the result needed to be more convincing. I started percutaneous hydrotomy sessions in mid-February. After each session, I felt a rebound, that is to say, a reaction of my antibodies because they were stimulated. The rebounds were less and less intense as the sessions progressed. After six sessions of abdominal mesovaccination (once per week), my eczema had disappeared entirely. I had smooth, solid, clear skin again. Happily, I stopped all my creams which never helped my condition. Since then, I felt like I'd gotten rid of a weight that I constantly carried. My immune defenses have strengthened; I don't even catch minor colds anymore! I am delighted with the result. I am cured! Knowing that I am not the only one to have suffered, I share my experience with great pleasure so that it can be helpful to others. Many thanks for the hydrotomy and mesovaccination. I certify that this testimony is accurate and sincere.

Mr. M., twenty-one years old, allergies and asthma, mesovaccination
Before the percutaneous hydrotomy treatments, I had two types of allergies: food and environmental. The food allergies caused my throat to swell and trigger asthma attacks. The environmental allergies (pollen, grasses, dust mites) triggered asthma attacks, swollen eyes, and runny noses. I took cortisone and an antihistamine all

Giving the Floor to the Patients: Testimonials

year round. In addition, I used two or three tubes of Ventolin [albuterol] per month for eight months of the year, from spring to fall. In mid-November 2018, I started mesovaccination injections. I had twelve injections. Today, I no longer have asthma. I no longer have an allergic reaction to pollen and dust mites. Asthma attacks started to decrease after the sixth session. After the eighth session, the allergies stopped. I work in the municipality of my village as a road worker, and I would never have been able to work a year ago with allergies. Without asthma, I can now play sports again, which was impossible for me.

Madame D., eighty-three years old, bronchitis, mesovaccination
Every year, I had two to three very severe bouts of bronchitis, often requiring long treatments with antibiotics, injections, oxygen, and even hospitalization. In December 2018, I was offered a mesovaccination protocol, one weekly session for three weeks, then monthly for three months. Since then, I no longer cough, it's the first winter I have spent without bronchitis, and I breathe much better.

Mr. P., seventy-nine years old, allergies, mesovaccination
It was at the beginning of 1968 (when I was living in Antibes) that I had my first purulent bronchitis/sinusitis. I was then treated with antibiotic drugs. At the beginning of 1970, faced with the aggravation of my condition, my general practitioner advised me to be treated by an ENT specialist (from Nice). He diagnosed that my problems were due to allergies. The treatments prescribed were always antibiotic-based, but the nasal breathing difficulties (nasal obstruction and severe discharge) did not improve. In February 1974, I underwent an urgent operation to correct a severe nasal

Stopping Pain

deviation. This improved, but my problems returned the following year, in the spring of 1975 (while we were living in Vence)—sinus infections, sneezing attacks, obstruction, runny nose, and bronchitis. My treatments were based on antibiotics, corticosteroid injections, and antihistamines. During the spring, I could only breathe using a cortisone-based inhaler. In 1985, the tests highlighted my allergy to cypress pollen. In the spring of 1986, my treatments were still based on corticosteroids. My doctor continued to treat me with antibiotics and antihistamines. Faced with the non-improvement of my condition, he often told me that one day I would meet the miracle doctor. It must be said that, during these thirty-two years, my wife, whom I thank very much for her help, and I have been through hell because very often, during heavy pollination, I didn't sleep for entire nights.

It was in mid-February 2001 that I met Dr. Bernard Guez in Nice. He then gave me the first mesovaccination session, and my allergic reactions immediately slowed down. He gave me a total of seven weekly sessions, and following the last session, I stopped all my treatments, including the inhalers. Since 2001, following my meeting with the miracle doctor (as predicted by my ENT doctor), my wife and I have resumed our lives, and my allergic problems have disappeared, and I still return for treatment as needed.

Irritable Bowel Syndrome (IBS) and Crohn's Disease

Mr. S., forty-six years old, irritable bowel syndrome, mesovaccination
Having irritable colon since my childhood, I am often subject to bloating and abdominal pain episodes. Without an identified cause and trying to pay attention to my diet, the symptoms persisted, and I decided to try abdominal mesovaccination. It's been a month since I started, and so far, there have been no episodes of bloating. In the

Giving the Floor to the Patients: Testimonials

same way, I intend to try to treat my gastric pains. I'm also being treated for neck pain, and currently, after six weeks of injections, I have experienced a regression of the symptoms.

Autoimmune Diseases

Miss T., twenty-five years old, rheumatoid disease, mesovaccination
I have had arthritis since I was two years old. It was silent until the end of high school, when the disease woke me up, attacking my right hip. Then in 2017, it attacked my right knee. A naturopath advised me of percutaneous hydrotomy. I started these sessions at the end of June 2018 with mesovaccination plus hydrotomy sessions on the knee. At the same time, I started basic treatment with methotrexate at the end of July. I also did chiropractic sessions. Before starting these sessions, I had a lot of pain, no strength, and walked abnormally. I also had mesoperfusion sessions for the hip. Today, I walk much better, and above all, I hardly think about my illness anymore.

CHAPTER 10

How to Find a Clinic and Common Questions

Patients often ask how they can find healthcare providers who offer percutaneous hydrotomy treatments. Since percutaneous hydrotomy is mainly available in Europe, it's relatively easy to find a practitioner there. In the United States, the technique is just starting to take off and it is much more difficult to find someone. Many doctors and health professionals are being trained in the technique. Please reach out to the ISPH about the possibility of finding a healthcare provider. Also, consider giving your healthcare provider this book. The techniques presented in this book are relatively simple to those who are accustomed to performing medical procedures. Those healthcare providers who are proficient in percutaneous techniques and surgical procedures are especially well adapted to performing regenerative techniques such as percutaneous hydrotomy.

The main hurdle for healthcare professionals to accept percutaneous hydrotomy is the understanding of how it works and how simple it is to perform. Since it is not covered by health insurance, the financial burden makes it difficult for both the healthcare provider and the patient. Below are some common questions that arise.

What is regenerative medicine?

Regenerative medicine (orthobiolologics) is an interdisciplinary field of medicine that addresses the underlying root causes of injuries and pain, not just the outward symptoms. Regenerative medicine procedures work by activating the healing processes our bodies naturally go through when we are injured, or not in homeostasis. Recognized regenerative medical techniques are prolotherapy, PRP, stem cell treatments, perineural injection therapy, saline injections, mesotherapy, percutaneous hydrotomy, and other related techniques.

What is percutaneous hydrotomy?

Percutaneous hydrotomy is a regenerative procedure where physiological saline, minerals, vitamins, amino acids, anti-inflammatories, chelating agents, local anesthetics, and medications are used to address the underlying cause of chronic diseases at the cellular level. It's the culmination of regenerative injection techniques, mesotherapy, water, oligotherapy, hypodermoclysis, and tumescent anesthesia. Percutaneous hydrotomy works by activating the healing processes and giving the cells the products needed to heal and become whole again. Percutaneous hydrotomy has been practiced for more than thirty years and over one million procedures have been performed.

A disclaimer for percutaneous hydrotomy

We're often asked what percutaneous hydrotomy is and where it fits into the treatment spectrum. First and foremost, it is neither a universal solution nor a miracle. The best way to think about all

Stopping Pain

this is in regard to the options you have with certain maladies. For example, if you have a severe corneal abrasion, which is a scratch on the eye's surface that can cause intense pain and potential infection, in most cases it should be treated with antibiotic eye drops and possibly a protective patch to promote healing and prevent complications. In this sense, there aren't many options.

But when you have a chronic disease like neck pain or migraines, many treatment options exist. It may be that you start with a consultation and start with physical therapy and taking an anti-inflammatory for osteoarthritis. Then, if the problem persists, you can consider other treatment modalities such as regenerative injection therapies discussed in this book. To reiterate, percutaneous hydrotomy is just another treatment that can help. In some cases, it will treat the chronic pain, and that is all you'll need to do. For others, it's a temporary solution until the time is right to consider surgery. It's important to speak with your healthcare provider and explore the best options.

Who's a good candidate for percutaneous hydrotomy?

Patients with chronic pain or musculoskeletal injuries who have not responded to conventional medicine, or are motivated to try other modalities to treat their pain or injuries, are good candidates for this type of treatment. For example, if neck or back pain has not responded to conventional modalities after three months, consider trying percutaneous hydrotomy or other regenerative procedures.

How many percutaneous hydrotomy sessions are usually needed?

Depending on the nature of the problem, one treatment may be enough to see positive results. A follow-up appointment is scheduled some weeks after each treatment, where the rehabilitation program is discussed further. In principle, most people experience some pain relief after the first treatment. For percutaneous hydrotomy to be effective long term, three to six treatments are usually prescribed.

Is there a recovery period after a percutaneous hydrotomy treatment?

Patients may experience discomfort for a couple of hours after treatment, but this pain subsides and is mild and controllable. The hydrotomy solution injected into the subcutaneous tissues resolves in about two hours. We advise patients to take it easy after the procedure and let the body rest.

Is percutaneous hydrotomy painful?

In general, it is not. However, it does involve an injection with a tiny needle. These needles can be seen in chapter 6. Once the diluted local anesthesia is placed over the area of concern, most patients experience no pain. It's also possible to apply ice and other modalities to numb the skin before an injection.

How long does a session for percutaneous hydrotomy last?

Hydrotomy using the hand-syringe technique takes about ten to thirty minutes, depending on the site(s) injected. Mesoperfusion can last from thirty to ninety minutes. Depending on what area is being treated, there's a lot of individual variation.

What is the price per treatment?

The price of percutaneous hydrotomy treatments varies depending on the technique used and the disease's complexity. Furthermore, the treatment is not the only thing included in the price—the healthcare practitioner's expertise, office space, supplies, prescriptive authority, and knowing when to refer a patient to a higher level of care are all things that go into providing the best care to patients.

Is there an organization that certifies practitioners of percutaneous hydrotomy?

Yes. The International Society of Percutaneous Hydrotomy (ISPH) provides training and education for practitioners. The courses are held in French currently under the direction of Dr. Bernard Guez in France. However, this is changing rapidly. Please contact the ISPH (www.percutaneoushydrotomy.net) for more opportunities to be trained in percutaneous hydrotomy.

Is percutaneous hydrotomy a temporary or durable treatment?

In principle, we must treat the underlying issues. Osteoarthritis most often represents a degenerative state, and the therapy must correct the imbalance. We do not seek to mask the pain symptoms using anti-inflammatory drugs (although their microcirculatory, antiplatelet, and blood-thinning effects are harnessed in this precise context) or analgesics. Instead, we aim to provide a regenerative treatment dealing with the underlying causes. Pain should not be masked to ensure a lasting effect. Moreover, the treatment has a long-lived effect.

Are maintenance sessions necessary?

Yes, maintenance sessions are occasionally appropriate, but the effects may decrease over time. In chronic osteoarthritis, maintenance sessions also help combat degeneration. We find that when percutaneous hydrotomy helps patients with chronic low back or knee pain, maintenance sessions are often necessary.

Does the ISPH advocate the use of Quinton plasma?

Quinton plasma is unsuitable for percutaneous hydrotomy because it does not have market authorization or FDA clearance for injections.

Is percutaneous hydrotomy the same as prolotherapy?

No, it is not, but similarities exist. Both involve subcutaneous injections of sterile water under the skin. But percutaneous hydrotomy goes further in providing the cells with minerals, vitamins, and certain medications to heal the cells causing the pathology. That being said, prolotherapy certainly has its advantages in treating many chronic diseases.

What evidence is there that there's any validity to percutaneous hydrotomy?

Studies are ongoing and have been presented in the United States, Africa, and Europe. A study on percutaneous hydrotomy in the treatment of low back pain was recently presented at the 50th Annual Regional Anesthesiology and Acute Pain Medicine Meeting in Orlando, Florida. We can attest to the benefits of percutaneous hydrotomy from our experiences of hundreds of thousands of procedures performed on thousands of patients. Apart from anecdotal evidence, our data comes from the literature, attending conferences, courses, and the numerous healthcare practitioners who practice the technique in over twenty-five countries. The data we have is of course not perfect, and neither is any data from orthopedic or pain medicine literature, for example. We often review and change our practice of medicine according to newer literature and patient outcomes. It should also be noted that conducting a study showing the effectiveness of a technique like percutaneous hydrotomy costs hundreds of thousands of dollars. The example of

Stopping Pain

prolotherapy is relevant. Even after millions of dollars were spent on level 1 studies showing that prolotherapy is effective, insurance companies still refuse to cover the cost of the treatment. This is all outlined in the book *Regenerative Healing for Life* by Dr. Brian Shiple. At the end of the day, healthcare professionals must make the best treatment choices for our patients to achieve the best outcome. Cutting-edge doctors still rely on case reports and case series to find new techniques.

References

Chapter One

Abate, Michele, Luigi Di Carlo, Sandra Verna, Patrizia Di Gregorio, Cosima Schiavone, and Vincenzo Salini. "Synergistic Activity of Platelet Rich Plasma and High Volume Image Guided Injection for Patellar Tendinopathy." *Knee Surgery, Sports Traumatology, Arthroscopy* 26, no. 12 (2018): 3645–51. https://doi.org/10.1007/s00167-018-4930-6.

Abramson, John. *Sickening: How Big Pharma Broke American Health Care and How We Can Repair It.* Mariner Books, 2023.

Acosta-Olivo, Carlos Alberto, Juan Manuel Millán-Alanís, Luis Ernesto Simental-Mendía, Neri Álvarez-Villalobos, Félix Vilchez-Cavazos, Víctor Manuel Peña-Martínez, and Mario Simental-Mendía. "Effect of Normal Saline Injections on Lateral Epicondylitis Symptoms: A Systematic Review and Meta-Analysis of Randomized Clinical Trials." *The American Journal of Sports Medicine* 48, no. 12 (2020): 3094–3102. https://doi.org/10.1177/0363546519899644.

Altman, Roy D., Tahira Devji, Mohit Bhandari, Anke Fierlinger, Faizan Niazi, and Robin Christensen. "Clinical Benefit of Intra-Articular Saline as a Comparator in Clinical Trials of Knee Osteoarthritis Treatments: A Systematic Review and Meta-Analysis of Randomized Trials." *Seminars in Arthritis and Rheumatism* 46, no. 2 (2016): 151–59. https://doi.org/10.1016/j.semarthrit.2016.04.003.

Stopping Pain

Billat, Veronique, and Johnathan Edwards. *Science of the Marathon and the Art of Variable Pace Running*. Tailwind Publications / Streetlight Graphics, 2020.

Cacchio, Angelo, Elisabetta De Blasis, Piergiorgio Desiati, Giorgio Spacca, Valter Santilli, and Fosco De Paulis. "Effectiveness of Treatment of Calcific Tendinitis of the Shoulder by Disodium EDTA." *Arthritis Care & Research* 61, no. 1 (2008): 84–91. https://doi.org/10.1002/art.24370.

Calavitta, Sam, and Monica Calavitta. *Making a Difference: Award Winning Math Teacher Changes the World One Student at a Time*. Shumway Publishing, 2010.

Edwards, Johnathan, and Gavin de Becker. *The Revolutionary Ketamine: The Safe Drug That Effectively Treats Depression and Prevents Suicide*. Skyhorse Publishing, 2023.

Gao, Burke, Shashank Dwivedi, Steven DeFroda, Steven Bokshan, Lauren V. Ready, Brian J. Cole, and Brett D. Owens. "The Therapeutic Benefits of Saline Solution Injection for Lateral Epicondylitis: A Meta-Analysis of Randomized Controlled Trials Comparing Saline Injections with Nonsurgical Injection Therapies." *Arthroscopy: The Journal of Arthroscopic & Related Surgery* 35, no. 6 (2019). https://doi.org/10.1016/j.arthro.2019.02.051.

Gazendam, Aaron, Seper Ekhtiari, Anthony Bozzo, Mark Phillips, and Mohit Bhandari. "Intra-Articular Saline Injection Is as Effective as Corticosteroids, Platelet-Rich Plasma and Hyaluronic Acid for Hip Osteoarthritis Pain: A Systematic Review and Network Meta-Analysis of Randomised Controlled Trials." *British Journal of Sports Medicine* 55, no. 5 (2020): 256–61. https://doi.org/10.1136/bjsports-2020-102179.

Guez, Bernard. *Vaincres Les Maladies Chronique Par L'hydrotomie Percutanee*. Dauphin Editions, 2021.

Linnanmäki, Lasse, Kari Kanto, Teemu Karjalainen, Olli V. Leppänen, and Janne Lehtinen. "Platelet-Rich Plasma or Autologous Blood Do Not Reduce Pain or Improve Function in Patients with Lateral Epicondylitis: A Randomized Controlled Trial." *Clinical Orthopaedics & Related Research* 478, no. 8 (2020): 1892–1900. https://doi.org/10.1097/corr.0000000000001185.

References

Mammucari, Massimo, Enrica Maggiori, Domenico Russo, Chiara Giorgio, Gianpaolo Ronconi, Paola E Ferrara, Flora Canzona, et al. "Mesotherapy: From Historical Notes to Scientific Evidence and Future Prospects." *Scientific World Journal* 2020 (2020): 1–9. https://doi.org/10.1155/2020/3542848.

Marquez-Lara, Alejandro, Ian D. Hutchinson, Fiesky Nuñez, Thomas L. Smith, and Anna N. Miller. "Nonsteroidal Anti-Inflammatory Drugs and Bone-Healing." *JBJS Reviews* 4, no. 3 (2016). https://doi.org/10.2106/jbjs.rvw.o.00055.

Olympics.com. "'Magic Man' David Taylor wins thriller to clinch Olympic title." August 5, 2021. https://olympics.com/en/news/david-taylor-begins-olympic-wrestling-campaign-with-bang.

Pitzurra, M., and P. Marconi. "Immunogenesis and Mesotherapy: The Immunoresponse to Antigens Inoculated Intradermally." *Giornale di Mesoterapia* 1 (1981): 9–14.

Pollack, Gerald H. *The Fourth Phase of Water: Beyond Solid, Liquid, and Vapor*. Ebner & Sons, 2013.

Previtali, Davide, Giulia Merli, Giorgio Di Laura Frattura, Christian Candrian, Stefano Zaffagnini, and Giuseppe Filardo. "The Long-Lasting Effects of 'Placebo Injections' in Knee Osteoarthritis: A Meta-Analysis." *CARTILAGE* 13, no. 1 suppl (2020). https://doi.org/10.1177/1947603520906597.

Prioux, France, Magali Barbieri, and Paul Reeve. "Recent Demographic Developments in France: Relatively Low Mortality at Advanced Ages." *Population* (English Edition) 67, no. 4 (2012): 493. https://doi.org/10.3917/pope.1204.0493.

Saltzman, Bryan M., Timothy Leroux, Maximilian A. Meyer, Bryce A. Basques, Jaskarndip Chahal, Bernard R. Bach, Adam B. Yanke, and Brian J. Cole. "The Therapeutic Effect of Intra-Articular Normal Saline Injections for Knee Osteoarthritis: A Meta-Analysis of Evidence Level 1 Studies." *The American Journal of Sports Medicine* 45, no. 11 (2016): 2647–53. https://doi.org/10.1177/0363546516680607.

Shipley, Brian J., and Marlise Wind. *Regenerative Healing for Life: A New Paradigm to Treat Injuries and Pain Without Surgery*. BookBaby, 2013.

Stopping Pain

Simental-Mendía, Mario, Félix Vilchez-Cavazos, Neri Álvarez-Villalobos, Jaime Blázquez-Saldaña, Víctor Peña-Martínez, Gregorio Villarreal-Villarreal, and Carlos Acosta-Olivo. "Clinical Efficacy of Platelet-Rich Plasma in the Treatment of Lateral Epicondylitis: A Systematic Review and Meta-Analysis of Randomized Placebo-Controlled Clinical Trials." *Clinical Rheumatology* 39, no. 8 (2020): 2255–65. https://doi.org/10.1007/s10067-020-05000-y.

Simon, Jolene M. "The Explosion of Complementary and Alternative Therapies." *International Journal of Nursing Terminologies and Classifications* 10, no. 3 (1999): 91–91. https://doi.org/10.1111/j.1744-618x.1999.tb00033.x.

Simonetta, Roberto, Arcangelo Russo, Michelangelo Palco, Giuseppe Gianluca Costa, and Pier Paolo Mariani. "Meniscus Tears Treatment: The Good, the Bad and the Ugly—Patterns Classification and Practical Guide." *World Journal of Orthopedics* 14, no. 4 (2023): 171–85. https://doi.org/10.5312/wjo.v14.i4.171.

Szent-Györgyi, Albert. *The Living State: With Observations On Cancer*. Academic Press, 1972.

Vora, Ariana, Joanne Borg-Stein, and Rosalyn T. Nguyen. "Regenerative Injection Therapy for Osteoarthritis: Fundamental Concepts and Evidence-Based Review." *PM&R* 4 (2012). https://doi.org/10.1016/j.pmrj.2012.02.005.

West, William, H., MD; Anthony I. Beutler, MD; and Christopher R. Gordon, MD, Abate, Michele, Luigi Di Carlo, Sandra Verna, Patrizia Di Gregorio, Cosima Schiavone, and Vincenzo Salini. "Synergistic Activity of Platelet Rich Plasma and High Volume Image Guided Injection for Patellar Tendinopathy." *Knee Surgery, Sports Traumatology, Arthroscopy* 26, no. 12 (2018): 3645–51. https://doi.org/10.1007/s00167-018-4930-6.

Williams SN, ML Wolford, and A Bercovitz. "Hospitalization for Total Knee Replacement Among Inpatients Aged 45 and Over: United States, 2000-2010." *NCHS Data Brief*. August 2015; (210):1–8. PMID: 26375255.

Yelland, Michael J., Paul P. Glasziou, Nikolai Bogduk, Philip J. Schluter, and Mary McKernon. "Prolotherapy Injections, Saline Injections, and Exercises for Chronic Low-Back Pain: A Randomized Trial." *Spine* 29, no. 1 (2004): 9–16. https://doi.org/10.1097/01.brs.0000105529.07222.5b.

References

Zelaya, CE. "Products—Data Briefs—Number 390—November 2020." Centers for Disease Control and Prevention, November 4, 2020. https://www.cdc.gov/nchs/products/databriefs/db390.htm.

Chapter 2

Abramson, John. *Sickening: How Big Pharma Broke American Health Care and How We Can Repair It*. Mariner Books, 2023.

Amerling, Richard. "COVID-19 Response Demonstrates the Tyranny of Evidence-Based Medicine." *Journal of American Physicians and Surgeons* 26, no. 4 (Winter 2021): 119–21.

Ansah, John P., and Chi-Tsun Chiu. "Projecting the Chronic Disease Burden among the Adult Population in the United States Using a Multi-State Population Model." *Frontiers in Public Health* 10 (2023). https://doi.org/10.3389/fpubh.2022.1082183.

Becker, Robert O. *The Body Electric: Electromagnetism and the Foundation Of Life*. William Morrow, 2020.

Bernell, Stephanie, and Steven W. Howard. "Use Your Words Carefully: What Is a Chronic Disease?" *Frontiers in Public Health* 4 (2016). https://doi.org/10.3389/fpubh.2016.00159.

Brownlee, Shannon. *Overtreated: Why Too Much Medicine Is Making Us Sicker and Poorer*. Bloomsbury, 2008.

Brune, K., B. Renner, and G. Tiegs. "Acetaminophen/Paracetamol: A History of Errors, Failures and False Decisions." *European Journal of Pain* 19, no. 7 (2014): 953–65. https://doi.org/10.1002/ejp.621.

Brunner-La Rocca, Hans-Peter, Lutz Fleischhacker, Olga Golubnitschaja, Frank Heemskerk, Thomas Helms, Thom Hoedemakers, Sandra Huygen Allianses, et al. "Challenges in Personalised Management of Chronic Diseases—Heart Failure as Prominent Example to Advance the Care Process." *EPMA Journal* 7, no. 1 (2015). https://doi.org/10.1186/s13167-016-0051-9.

Carlson, Hans, and Nels Carlson. "An Overview of the Management of Persistent Musculoskeletal Pain." *Therapeutic Advances in Musculoskeletal Disease* 3, no. 2 (2011): 91–99. https://doi.org/10.1177/1759720x11398742.

Stopping Pain

CDC. 2022. "Products—Vital Statistics Rapid Release—Provisional Drug Overdose Data." CDC. 2022. https://www.cdc.gov/nchs/nvss/vsrr/drug-overdose-data.htm.

Erren, Thomas C., Peter Morfeld, J. Valérie Groß, Ursula Wild, and Philip Lewis. "IARC 2019: 'Night Shift Work' Is Probably Carcinogenic: What about Disturbed Chronobiology in All Walks of Life?" *Journal of Occupational Medicine and Toxicology* 14, no. 1 (2019). https://doi.org/10.1186/s12995-019-0249-6.

Ferreira, Manuela L., Katie de Luca, Lydia M. Haile, Jaimie D. Steinmetz, Garland T. Culbreth, Marita Cross, Jacek A. Kopec, et al. "Global, Regional, and National Burden of Low Back Pain, 1990–2020, Its Attributable Risk Factors, and Projections to 2050: A Systematic Analysis of the Global Burden of Disease Study 2021." *The Lancet Rheumatology* 5, no. 6 (2023). https://doi.org/10.1016/s2665-9913(23)00098-x.

Garber, Judith, and Shannon Brownlee. "Medication Overload: America's Other Drug Problem." 2019. https://doi.org/10.46241/li.wouk3548.

Guez, Bernard. *Vaincres Les Maladies Chronique Par L'hydrotomie Percutanee.* Dauphin Editions, 2021.

Haenisch, Britta, Klaus von Holt, Birgitt Wiese, Jana Prokein, Carolin Lange, Annette Ernst, Christian Brettschneider, et al. "Risk of Dementia in Elderly Patients with the Use of Proton Pump Inhibitors." *European Archives of Psychiatry and Clinical Neuroscience* 265, no. 5 (2014): 419–28. https://doi.org/10.1007/s00406-014-0554-0.

Heying, Heather, and Bret Weinstein. *A Hunter-Gatherer's Guide to the 21st Century: Evolution and the Challenges of Modern Life.* Swift Press, 2022.

Hippisley-Cox, Julia, and Carol Coupland. "Risk of Myocardial Infarction in Patients Taking Cyclo-Oxygenase-2 Inhibitors or Conventional Non-Steroidal Anti-Inflammatory Drugs: Population Based Nested Case-Control Analysis." *BMJ* 330, no. 7504 (2005): 1366. https://doi.org/10.1136/bmj.330.7504.1366.

Holman, Halsted R. "The Relation of the Chronic Disease Epidemic to the Health Care Crisis." *ACR Open Rheumatology* 2, no. 3 (2020): 167–73. https://doi.org/10.1002/acr2.11114.

References

Ibeanu, Vivienne N., Chinonye G. Edeh, and Peace N. Ani. "Evidence-Based Strategy for Prevention of Hidden Hunger among Adolescents in a Suburb of Nigeria." *BMC Public Health* 20, no. 1 (2020). https://doi.org/10.1186/s12889-020-09729-8.

Kau, Andrew L., Philip P. Ahern, Nicholas W. Griffin, Andrew L. Goodman, and Jeffrey I. Gordon. "Human Nutrition, the Gut Microbiome and the Immune System." *Nature* 474, no. 7351 (2011): 327–36. https://doi.org/10.1038/nature10213.

Kubitza, Jenny, Margit Haas, Lena Keppeler, and Bernd Reuschenbach. "Therapy Options for Those Affected by a Long Lie after a Fall: A Scoping Review." *BMC Geriatrics* 22, no. 1 (2022). https://doi.org/10.1186/s12877-022-03258-2.

Kuijpers, Suzanne M., Chantal M. Wiepjes, Elfi B. Conemans, Alessandra D. Fisher, Guy T'Sjoen, and Martin den Heijer. "Toward a Lowest Effective Dose of Cyproterone Acetate in Trans Women: Results from the ENIGI Study." *The Journal of Clinical Endocrinology & Metabolism* 106, no. 10 (2021). https://doi.org/10.1210/clinem/dgab427.

Lapeyre-Mestre, Maryse, Sabrina Grolleau, and Jean-Louis Montastruc. "Adverse Drug Reactions Associated with the Use of NSAIDs: A Case/Noncase Analysis of Spontaneous Reports from the French Pharmacovigilance Database 2002–2006." *Fundamental & Clinical Pharmacology* 27, no. 2 (2011): 223–30. https://doi.org/10.1111/j.1472-8206.2011.00991.x.

Larson, Anne M., Julie Polson, Robert J. Fontana, Timothy J. Davern, Ezmina Lalani, Linda S. Hynan, Joan S. Reisch, et al. "Acetaminophen-Induced Acute Liver Failure: Results of a United States Multicenter, Prospective Study." *Hepatology* 42, no. 6 (2005): 1364–72. https://doi.org/10.1002/hep.20948.

Leopoldino, Amanda O., Gustavo C. Machado, Paulo H. Ferreira, Marina B. Pinheiro, Richard Day, Andrew J. McLachlan, David J. Hunter, and Manuela L. Ferreira. "Paracetamol versus Placebo for Knee and Hip Osteoarthritis." *Cochrane Database of Systematic Reviews* 2019, no. 8 (2019). https://doi.org/10.1002/14651858.cd013273.

Stopping Pain

Maté, Gabor, and Daniel Maté. *The Myth of Normal: Trauma, Illness and Healing in a Toxic Culture.* Vintage Canada, 2023.

Mauck, Matthew C., Jeffrey Lotz, Matthew A. Psioda, Timothy S. Carey, Daniel J. Clauw, Sharmila Majumdar, William S. Marras, et al. "The Back Pain Consortium (Bacpac) Research Program: Structure, Research Priorities, and Methods." *Pain Medicine* 24, no. Supplement 1 (2023). https://doi.org/10.1093/pm/pnac202.

Mills, Sarah E. E., Karen P. Nicolson, and Blair H. Smith. "Chronic Pain: A Review of Its Epidemiology and Associated Factors in Population-Based Studies." *British Journal of Anaesthesia* 123, no. 2 (2019). https://doi.org/10.1016/j.bja.2019.03.023.

Muscat, Joshua E. "Handheld Cellular Telephone Use and Risk of Brain Cancer." *JAMA* 284, no. 23 (2000): 3001. https://doi.org/10.1001/jama.284.23.3001.

Ortiz-Guerrero, Gloria, Diana Amador-Muñoz, Carlos Alberto Calderón-Ospina, Daniel López-Fuentes, and Mauricio Orlando Nava Mesa. "Proton Pump Inhibitors and Dementia: Physiopathological Mechanisms and Clinical Consequences." *Neural Plasticity* 2018 (2018): 1–9. https://doi.org/10.1155/2018/5257285.

Prakash, Snigdha, and Vikki Valentine. "Timeline: The Rise and Fall of Vioxx." NPR, November 10, 2007. https://www.npr.org/2007/11/10/5470430/timeline-the-rise-and-fall-of-vioxx.

Radawski, Christine, Mark C. Genovese, Brett Hauber, W. Benjamin Nowell, Kelly Hollis, Carol L. Gaich, Amy M. DeLozier, et al. "Patient Perceptions of Unmet Medical Need in Rheumatoid Arthritis: A Cross-Sectional Survey in the USA." *Rheumatology and Therapy* 6, no. 3 (2019): 461–71. https://doi.org/10.1007/s40744-019-00168-5.

SeaWeb. "Chemicals In Our Waters Are Affecting Humans And Aquatic Life In Unanticipated Ways." *ScienceDaily*, February 21, 2008. www.sciencedaily.com/releases/2008/02/080216095740.htm

Shi, Hongying, Tianyi Huang, Eva S. Schernhammer, Qi Sun, and Molin Wang. "Rotating Night Shift Work and Healthy Aging after 24 Years of Follow-up in the Nurses' Health Study." *JAMA Network Open* 5, no. 5 (2022). https://doi.org/10.1001/jamanetworkopen.2022.10450.

References

Vos, Theo, Amanuel Alemu Abajobir, Kalkidan Hassen Abate, Cristiana Abbafati, Kaja M Abbas, Foad Abd-Allah, Rizwan Suliankatchi Abdulkader, et al. "Global, Regional, and National Incidence, Prevalence, and Years Lived with Disability for 328 Diseases and Injuries for 195 Countries, 1990–2016: A Systematic Analysis for the Global Burden of Disease Study 2016." *The Lancet* 390, no. 10100 (2017): 1211–59. https://doi.org/10.1016/s0140-6736(17)32154-2.

Wong, Stella Pui, and Chi Chiu Mok. "Management of Glucocorticoid-Related Osteoporotic Vertebral Fracture." *Osteoporosis and Sarcopenia* 6, no. 1 (2020): 1–7. https://doi.org/10.1016/j.afos.2020.02.002.

Zelaya, C. E. "Products—Data Briefs—Number 390—November 2020." Centers for Disease Control and Prevention, November 4, 2020. https://www.cdc.gov/nchs/products/databriefs/db390.htm.

Chapter 3

Adem, Sittelbenat, and Nabil Almouaalamy. "Effectiveness and Safety of Hypodermoclysis Patients with Cancer: A Single-Center Experience from Saudi Arabia." *Cureus*, 2021. https://doi.org/10.7759/cureus.13785.

"Administration of Fluids by Hypodermoclysis." *Journal of the American Medical Association* 150, no. 9 (1952): 942. https://doi.org/10.1001/jama.1952.03680090106014.

Altman, Roy D., Tahira Devji, Mohit Bhandari, Anke Fierlinger, Faizan Niazi, and Robin Christensen. "Clinical Benefit of Intra-Articular Saline as a Comparator in Clinical Trials of Knee Osteoarthritis Treatments: A Systematic Review and Meta-Analysis of Randomized Trials." *Seminars in Arthritis and Rheumatism* 46, no. 2 (2016): 151–59. https://doi.org/10.1016/j.semarthrit.2016.04.003.

"Practice Parameter: The Management of Acute Gastroenteritis in Young Children." *Pediatrics* 97, no. 3 (1996): 424–35. https://doi.org/10.1542/peds.97.3.424.

Berger, Eugene Y. "Nutrition by Hypodermoclysis." *Journal of the American Geriatrics Society* 32, no. 3 (1984): 199–203. https://doi.org/10.1111/j.1532-5415.1984.tb02002.x.

Stopping Pain

Bonnet, C., D. Laurens, and J. J. Perrin. *Practical Guide to Mesotherapy.* Elsevier-Masson, 2012.

"Book Review: Trace Elements in Human Nutrition and Health." *Nutrition and Health* 11, no. 2 (1996): 133–34. https://doi.org/10.1177/026010609601100206.

Bruno, Vanessa Galuppo. "Hypodermoclysis: A Literature Review to Assist in Clinical Practice." *Einstein* (São Paulo) 13, no. 1 (2015): 122–28. https://doi.org/10.1590/s1679-45082015rw2572.

Burford G. (1913). "Saline Injections in Infantile Diarrhœa." *The Hospital*, 54 (1414), 542 (1913).

D'alloz-Bourguignon, André. *Dix Gestes de mésothérapie [Ten Gestures of Mesotherapy].* Maloine, 1980.

Dardaine-Giraud, V., M. Lamandé, and T. Constans. "L'hypodermoclyse : Intérêts et Indications En Gériatrie." *La Revue de Médecine Interne* 26, no. 8 (2005): 643–50. https://doi.org/10.1016/j.revmed.2005.03.016.

Day, J. R., "Saline Injections in Infantile Diarrhœa." *Hospital* (London 1886). 1913 Jul 26; 54 (1413):512. PMID: 29828342; PMCID: PMC5243087.

Day, HB. "Saline Injections in Infantile Diarrhœa." *The Hospital* (Lond 1886) 54, no. 1413 (July 26, 1913): 512.

Farrand, S., and A. J. Campbell. "Safe, Simple Subcutaneous Fluid Administration." *Br J Hosp Med.* 1996 Jun 5–18;55(11):690–2. PMID: 8793132, 11, 18, no. 55 (June 5, 1996): 690–92. https://doi.org/PMID: 8793132.

Fortan. "Discours Prononcés Aux Obsèques de René Quinton Le 13 Juillet 1925." Gallica, January 1, 1970. https://gallica.bnf.fr/ark:/12148/bpt6k856814t?rk=171674%3B4.

Fournier, Pierre François. *Liposculpture: Ma Technique.* Arnette Blackwell, 1996.

Gao, Yue, Xia Li, Tao Liu, and Zheng Liu. "The Effect of Methotrexate on Serum Levels of Trace/Mineral Elements in Patients with Psoriatic Arthritis." *Biological Trace Element Research* 199, no. 12 (2021): 4498–4503. https://doi.org/10.1007/s12011-021-02594-5.

References

Giordano, C., N. L. Onyinyechi, and Sara, C. "Hypodermoclysis: The Modern Use in Care of an Ancient Therapeutic Technic." *J Hosp Palliat Med Care* 1: 003. (December 18, 2018).

Guez, Bernard. *Vaincres Les Maladies Chronique Par L'hydrotomie Percutanee.* Dauphin Editions, 2021.

Hanke, C., and Michael Dent. "Tumescent Anesthesia: A Brief History Regarding the Evolution of Tumescent Solution." *Journal of Drugs in Dermatology* 20, no. 12 (2021): 1283–87. https://doi.org/10.36849/jdd.6212.

Hartung, O., O. Creton, and S. Penillon. "Anesthésie Locale Par Tumescence." *Veines superficielles et profondes des membres*, 2023, 36–39. https://doi.org/10.1016/b978-2-294-77730-1.00004-1.

"Hypodermoclysis in Cholera." *Lancet* 126, no. 3249 (1885): 1058. https://doi.org/10.1016/s0140-6736(02)29118-7.

Imber, Gerald, and William Stewart Halsted. *Genius on the Edge: The Bizarre Double Life of Dr. William Stewart Halsted*. Kaplan Publishing, 2011.

"J. Jarricot. Le Dispensaire Marin. Un Organisme Nouveau de Puériculture.—Paris, Masson, 1921. In-80, 628 P., 54 Pl." *Revue Internationale de la Croix-Rouge et Bulletin international des Sociétés de la Croix-Rouge* 4, no. 42 (1922): 500. https://doi.org/10.1017/s1026881200014045.

Jet Propulsion Laboratory. "New Study Outlines 'Water World' Theory of Life's Origins." NASA, April 15, 2014. https://www.jpl.nasa.gov/news/new-study-outlines-water-world-theory-of-lifes-origins.

Klein, Jeffrey A. "Tumescent Technique for Local Anesthesia Improves Safety in Large-Volume Liposuction." *Plastic and Reconstructive Surgery* 92, no. 6 (1993): 1085–98. https://doi.org/10.1097/00006534-199311000-00014.

Koulakis, John P., Joshua Rouch, Nhan Huynh, Holden H. Wu, James C. Dunn, and Seth Putterman. "Tumescent Injections in Subcutaneous Pig Tissue Disperse Fluids Volumetrically and Maintain Elevated Local Concentrations of Additives for Several Hours, Suggesting a Treatment for Drug Resistant Wounds." *Pharmaceutical Research* 37, no. 3 (2020). https://doi.org/10.1007/s11095-020-2769-2.

Stopping Pain

Le Boutillier, Theodore. "Sea-Water Treatment, Given by Subcutaneous Injection." *Journal of the American Medical Association* LIV, no. 1 (1910): 26. https://doi.org/10.1001/jama.1910.92550270001001h.

Mammucari, Massimo, Enrica Maggiori, Domenico Russo, Chiara Giorgio, Gianpaolo Ronconi, Paola E. Ferrara, Flora Canzona, et al. "Mesotherapy: From Historical Notes to Scientific Evidence and Future Prospects." *Scientific World Journal* 2020 (2020): 1–9. https://doi.org/10.1155/2020/3542848.

Matarasso, Alan, and Tracy M. Pfeifer. "Mesotherapy and Injection Lipolysis." *Clinics in Plastic Surgery* 36, no. 2 (2009): 181–92. https://doi.org/10.1016/j.cps.2008.11.002.

Miller, Charles. "Intraperitoneal Saline Injections in Epidemic Diarrhœa." *Lancet* 182, no. 4697 (1913): 774. https://doi.org/10.1016/s0140-6736(01)77966-4.

Nielsen, Forrest H. "New Essential Trace Elements for the Life Sciences." *Nuclear Analytical Methods in the Life Sciences*, 1990, 599–611. https://doi.org/10.1007/978-1-4612-0473-2_65.

Norn, S, PR Kruse, and E Kruse. "Traek Af Injektionens Historie [On the History of Injection]." *Dan Medicinhist Arbog* 34 (2006): 104–13.

Picard, Henry. *Vaincre L'arthrose: La Découverte De La Cause Et Du Traitement De L'arthrose*. du Rocher, 2000.

Pistor, M. "Qu'est-Ce Que La Mésothérapie? [What Is Mesotherapy?]." *Chir Dent Fr.* 46, no. 288 (January 21, 1976): 59–60. https://doi.org/PMID: 1076080.

Pistor, Michel. *Mésothérapie Pratique*. Masson, 1998.

Pistor, Michel. *Un défi thérapeutique: La Mésothérapie*. Maloine, 1986.

Quinton, R. *L'Eau de Mer, Milieu Organique*. Masson et Cie, 1912.

Remington, Ruth, and Todd Hultman. "Hypodermoclysis to Treat Dehydration: A Review of the Evidence." *Journal of the American Geriatrics Society* 55, no. 12 (2007): 2051–55. https://doi.org/10.1111/j.1532-5415.2007.01437.x.

Renard. "Discours Prononcés Aux Obsèques de René Quinton Le 13 Juillet 1925." Gallica, January 1, 1970. https://gallica.bnf.fr/ark:/12148/bpt6k856814t?rk=171674%3B4.

References

Rondanelli, Mariangela, Milena Anna Faliva, Gabriella Peroni, Vittoria Infantino, Clara Gasparri, Giancarlo Iannello, Simone Perna, Antonella Riva, Giovanna Petrangolini, and Alice Tartara. "Pivotal Role of Boron Supplementation on Bone Health: A Narrative Review." *Journal of Trace Elements in Medicine and Biology* 62 (2020): 126577. https://doi.org/10.1016/j.jtemb.2020.126577.

Rotunda, A., et al. "Mesotherapy and Phosphatidylcholine Injections: Historical Clarification and Review." *Dermatologic Surgery* 32, no. 4 (2006): 465–80. https://doi.org/10.1111/j.1524-4725.2006.32100.x.

Rotunda, Adam M. "Mesotherapy and Injectable Lipolysis." *Facial Rejuvenation*, n.d., 147–65. https://doi.org/10.1007/978-3-540-69518-9_7.

Scott, Alex, Robert F. LaPrade, Kimberly G. Harmon, Giuseppe Filardo, Elizaveta Kon, Stefano Della Villa, Roald Bahr, et al. "Platelet-Rich Plasma for Patellar Tendinopathy: A Randomized Controlled Trial of Leukocyte-Rich PRP or Leukocyte-Poor PRP versus Saline." *The American Journal of Sports Medicine* 47, no. 7 (2019): 1654–61. https://doi.org/10.1177/0363546519837954.

Shipley, Brian J., and Marlise Wind. *Regenerative Healing for Life: A New Paradigm to Treat Injuries and Pain Without Surgery.* BookBaby, 2013.

Sivagnanam, G. "Mesotherapy—the French Connection." *Journal of Pharmacology and Pharmacotherapeutics* 1, no. 1 (2010): 4–8. https://doi.org/10.4103/0976-500x.64529.

Spandorfer, Philip R. "Subcutaneous Rehydration." *Pediatric Emergency Care* 27, no. 3 (2011): 230–36. https://doi.org/10.1097/pec.0b013e31820e1405.

Steiner, Nathalie, and Eduardo Bruera. "Methods of Hydration in Palliative Care Patients." *Journal of Palliative Care* 14, no. 2 (1998): 6–13. https://doi.org/10.1177/082585979801400202.

Welch, J. "History of Tumescent Anesthesia, Part I: From American Surgical Textbooks of the 1920s and 1930s." *Aesthetic Surgery Journal* 18, no. 5 (1998): 353–57. https://doi.org/10.1016/s1090-820x(98)70091-3.

Zhang, W., J. Robertson, A. C. Jones, P. A. Dieppe, and M. Doherty. "The Placebo Effect and Its Determinants in Osteoarthritis: Meta-Analysis of Randomised Controlled Trials." *Annals of the Rheumatic Diseases* 67, no. 12 (2008): 1716–23. https://doi.org/10.1136/ard.2008.092015.

Chapter 4

Breit, Sigrid, Aleksandra Kupferberg, Gerhard Rogler, and Gregor Hasler. "Vagus Nerve as Modulator of the Brain–Gut Axis in Psychiatric and Inflammatory Disorders." *Frontiers in Psychiatry* 9 (2018). https://doi.org/10.3389/fpsyt.2018.00044.

Dalloz-Bourguignon, André. *Dix Gestes de mésothérapie [Ten Gestures of Mesotherapy]*h. Maloine, 1980.

Denis, François, Sophie Alain, and Marie-Cécile Ploy. "Nouvelles Voies d'administration: Vaccinations Par Voie Épidermique, Intradermique, Muqueuse." *Médecine/Sciences* 23, no. 4 (2007): 379–85. https://doi.org/10.1051/medsci/2007234379.

Egunsola, Oluwaseun, Fiona Clement, John Taplin, Liza Mastikhina, Joyce W. Li, Diane L. Lorenzetti, Laura E. Dowsett, and Tom Noseworthy. "Immunogenicity and Safety of Reduced-Dose Intradermal vs Intramuscular Influenza Vaccines." *JAMA Network Open* 4, no. 2 (2021). https://doi.org/10.1001/jamanetworkopen.2020.35693.

Freitas Santoro, Dalton de, Luciene Barbosa de Sousa, Niels O. Câmara, Denise de Freitas, and Lauro Augusto de Oliveira. "SARS-COV-2 and Ocular Surface: From Physiology to Pathology, a Route to Understand Transmission and Disease." *Frontiers in Physiology* 12 (2021). https://doi.org/10.3389/fphys.2021.612319.

Guez, B. "Reflections on mesovaccination." Annual meeting of the International Society of Percutaneous Hydrotomy, 2021, Nice, France.

Henein, Michael Y., Sergio Vancheri, Giovanni Longo, and Federico Vancheri. "The Role of Inflammation in Cardiovascular Disease." *International Journal of Molecular Sciences* 23, no. 21 (2022): 12906. https://doi.org/10.3390/ijms232112906.

Jin, K. "Modern Biological Theories of Aging." *Aging and Disease* 1, no. 2 (August 1, 2010): 72–74.

Kenney, Richard T., Sarah A. Frech, Larry R. Muenz, Christina P. Villar, and Gregory M. Glenn. "Dose Sparing with Intradermal Injection of Influenza Vaccine." *New England Journal of Medicine* 351, no. 22 (2004): 2295–2301. https://doi.org/10.1056/nejmoa043540.

References

La Montagne, John R., and Anthony S. Fauci. "Intradermal Influenza Vaccination—Can Less Be More?" *New England Journal of Medicine* 351, no. 22 (2004): 2330–32. https://doi.org/10.1056/nejme048314.

Lefrancq, E., and F. Pittolo. "Reflections and results of the psychosomatic axis and its applications for cardiologists and psychologists." Annual meeting of the International Society of Percutaneous Hydrotomy, 2021, Nice, France.

Levine, Glenn N. "The Mind-Heart-Body Connection." *Circulation* 140, no. 17 (2019): 1363–65. https://doi.org/10.1161/circulationaha.119.041914.

Maeda, Kazuhiko, Matias J. Caldez, and Shizuo Akira. "Innate Immunity in Allergy." *Allergy* 74, no. 9 (2019): 1660–74. https://doi.org/10.1111/all.13788.

Marques, M. P., A. L. Batista de Carvalho, A. P. Mamede, A. Dopplapudi, V. García Sakai, and L. A. Batista de Carvalho. "Role of Intracellular Water in the Normal-to-Cancer Transition in Human Cells—Insights from Quasi-Elastic Neutron Scattering." *Structural Dynamics* 7, no. 5 (2020). https://doi.org/10.1063/4.0000021.

Marra, Fawziah, Flora Young, Kathryn Richardson, and Carlo A. Marra. "A Meta-Analysis of Intradermal versus Intramuscular Influenza Vaccines: Immunogenicity and Adverse Events." *Influenza and Other Respiratory Viruses* 7, no. 4 (2012): 584–603. https://doi.org/10.1111/irv.12000.

Morishita, Kazuhiro, Kengo Watanabe, and Hidenori Ichijo. "Cell Volume Regulation in Cancer Cell Migration Driven by Osmotic Water Flow." *Cancer Science* 110, no. 8 (2019): 2337–47. https://doi.org/10.1111/cas.14079.

Multedo, Jean-Pierre. *Mésothérapie: Les Dessous de la Peau*. BoD—Books on Demand, 2018.

Pahwa, R., A. Goyal, and I. Jialal. "Chronic Inflammation." StatPearls, August 8, 2022.

Picard, Henry. *Vaincre L'arthrose: La Découverte De La Cause Et Du Traitement De L'arthrose*. du Rocher, 2000.

Pistor, Michel. *Un Défi Thérapeutique: La Mésothérapie*. Maloine, 1986.

Pollack, Gerald H. *The Fourth Phase Of Water: Beyond Solid, Liquid, and Vapor*. Ebner & Sons, 2013

Stopping Pain

Shakouri, Alireza A., and Sami L. Bahna. "Hypersensitivity to Antihistamines." *Allergy and Asthma Proceedings* 34, no. 6 (2013): 488–96. https://doi.org/10.2500/aap.2013.34.3699.

Song, Joon Young, Hee Jin Cheong, Ji Yun Noh, Tae Un Yang, Yu Bin Seo, Kyung-Wook Hong, In Seon Kim, Won Suk Choi, and Woo Joo Kim. "Long-Term Immunogenicity of the Influenza Vaccine at Reduced Intradermal and Full Intramuscular Doses among Healthy Young Adults." *Clinical and Experimental Vaccine Research* 2, no. 2 (2013): 115. https://doi.org/10.7774/cevr.2013.2.2.115.

Szent-Györgyi, Albert. *The Living State: With Observations on Cancer.* Academic Press, 1972.

Timmerman, Kyle L, and Elena Volpi. "Amino Acid Metabolism and Regulatory Effects in Aging." *Current Opinion in Clinical Nutrition and Metabolic Care* 11, no. 1 (2008): 45–49. https://doi.org/10.1097/mco.0b013e3282f2a592.

Vaccarino, Viola, Amit J. Shah, Puja K. Mehta, Brad Pearce, Paolo Raggi, J. Douglas Bremner, and Arshed A. Quyyumi. "Brain-Heart Connections in Stress and Cardiovascular Disease: Implications for the Cardiac Patient." *Atherosclerosis* 328 (2021): 74–82. https://doi.org/10.1016/j.atherosclerosis.2021.05.020.

Chapter 5

Abate, M., Di Carlo, L., Verna, S., Di Gregorio, P., Schiavone, C., Salini, V. "Synergistic activity of platelet rich plasma and high volume image guided injection for patellar tendinopathy." *Knee Surg Sports Traumatol Arthrosc.* December 2018; 26 (12):3645-3651. doi: 10.1007/s00167-018-4930-6. Epub 2018 Mar 31. PMID: 29605861.

Acosta-Olivo, Carlos Alberto, Juan Manuel Millán-Alanís, Luis Ernesto Simental-Mendía, Neri Álvarez-Villalobos, Félix Vilchez-Cavazos, Víctor Manuel Peña-Martínez, and Mario Simental-Mendía. "Effect of Normal Saline Injections on Lateral Epicondylitis Symptoms: A Systematic Review and Meta-Analysis of Randomized Clinical Trials." *The American Journal of Sports Medicine* 48, no. 12 (2020): 3094–3102. https://doi.org/10.1177/0363546519899644.

References

Alexander, W. "Branko Furst's Radical Alternative: Is the Heart Moved by the Blood, Rather than Vice Versa?" *P & T* 42, no. 1 (2017): 33–39.

Altman, R., et al. "Clinical Benefit of Intra-Articular Saline as a Comparator in Clinical Trials of Knee Osteoarthritis Treatments: A Systematic Review and Meta-Analysis of Randomized Trials." *Seminars in Arthritis and Rheumatism* 46, no. 2 (2016): 151–59. https://doi.org/10.1016/j.semarthrit.2016.04.003.

Angelakis, Emmanouil. "Weight Gain by Gut Microbiota Manipulation in Productive Animals." *Microbial Pathogenesis* 106 (2017): 162–70. https://doi.org/10.1016/j.micpath.2016.11.002.

Bernard, Claude. *Leçons Sur Les Propriétés Physiologiques Et Les Altérations Pathologiques Des Liquides De L'organisme.* J.B. Baillee`re, 1977.

Breedlove, Byron, and J. Todd Weber. "'No Water, No Life. No Blue, No Green.'" *Emerging Infectious Diseases* 24, no. 4 (2018): 815–16. https://doi.org/10.3201/eid2404.ac2404.

Capozzi, A., G. Scambia, S. Migliaccio, and S. Lello. "Role of Vitamin K2 in Bone Metabolism: A Point of View and a Short Reappraisal of the Literature." *Gynecological Endocrinology* 36, no. 4 (2019): 285–88. https://doi.org/10.1080/09513590.2019.1689554.

Cody, GW. "The Origins of Integrative Medicine—The First True Integrators: The Roots." *Integrative Medicine* (Encinitas, Calif.) 17, no. 1 (February 2018): 18–21.

Debernardi, A. Etal. "Alcmaeon of Croton." *Neurosurgery* 66, no. 2 (2010): 247–52. https://doi.org/10.1227/01.neu.0000363193.24806.02.

Gao, Burke, Shashank Dwivedi, Steven DeFroda, Steven Bokshan, Lauren V. Ready, Brian J. Cole, and Brett D. Owens. "The Therapeutic Benefits of Saline Solution Injection for Lateral Epicondylitis: A Meta-Analysis of Randomized Controlled Trials Comparing Saline Injections with Nonsurgical Injection Therapies." *Arthroscopy: The Journal of Arthroscopic & Related Surgery* 35, no. 6 (2019). https://doi.org/10.1016/j.arthro.2019.02.051.

Gasser, Tobias M., Alexander V. Thoeny, A. Dominic Fortes, and Thomas Loerting. "Structural Characterization of Ice XIX as the Second

Polymorph Related to ICE VI." *Nature Communications* 12, no. 1 (2021). https://doi.org/10.1038/s41467-021-21161-z.

Gazendam, Aaron, Seper Ekhtiari, Anthony Bozzo, Mark Phillips, and Mohit Bhandari. "Intra-Articular Saline Injection Is as Effective as Corticosteroids, Platelet-Rich Plasma and Hyaluronic Acid for Hip Osteoarthritis Pain: A Systematic Review and Network Meta-Analysis of Randomised Controlled Trials." *British Journal of Sports Medicine* 55, no. 5 (2020): 256–61. https://doi.org/10.1136/bjsports-2020-102179.

Gupta, Ramesh C., Rajiv Lall, Ajay Srivastava, and Anita Sinha. "Hyaluronic Acid: Molecular Mechanisms and Therapeutic Trajectory." *Frontiers in Veterinary Science* 6 (2019). https://doi.org/10.3389/fvets.2019.00192.

Hall, John E., and Michael E. Hall. *Guyton and Hall Textbook of Medical Physiology*. Elsevier, 2021.

Hanke, W., et al. "Tumescent Liposuction Report Performance Measurement Initiative." *Dermatologic Surgery* 30, no. 7 (2004): 967–77. https://doi.org/10.1097/00042728-200407000-00001.

Hussain, Md. Saddam, and Tanoy Mazumder. "Long-Term Use of Proton Pump Inhibitors Adversely Affects Minerals and Vitamin Metabolism, Bone Turnover, Bone Mass, and Bone Strength." *Journal of Basic and Clinical Physiology and Pharmacology* 33, no. 5 (2021): 567–79. https://doi.org/10.1515/jbcpp-2021-0203.

Jahn, Sabrina, Jasmine Seror, and Jacob Klein. "Lubrication of Articular Cartilage." *Annual Review of Biomedical Engineering* 18, no. 1 (2016): 235–58. https://doi.org/10.1146/annurev-bioeng-081514-123305.

Jéquier, E, and F Constant. "Water as an Essential Nutrient: The Physiological Basis of Hydration." *European Journal of Clinical Nutrition* 64, no. 2 (2009): 115–23. https://doi.org/10.1038/ejcn.2009.111.

Kau, Andrew L., Philip P. Ahern, Nicholas W. Griffin, Andrew L. Goodman, and Jeffrey I. Gordon. "Human Nutrition, the Gut Microbiome and the Immune System." *Nature* 474, no. 7351 (2011): 327–36. https://doi.org/10.1038/nature10213.

Koulakis, John P., Joshua Rouch, Nhan Huynh, Holden H. Wu, James C. Dunn, and Seth Putterman. "Tumescent Injections in Subcutaneous Pig Tissue Disperse Fluids Volumetrically and Maintain Elevated Local

References

Concentrations of Additives for Several Hours, Suggesting a Treatment for Drug Resistant Wounds." *Pharmaceutical Research* 37, no. 3 (2020). https://doi.org/10.1007/s11095-020-2769-2.

Kundacina, Nenad, Minghui Shi, and Gerald H. Pollack. "Effect of Local and General Anesthetics on Interfacial Water." *PLOS-ONE* 11, no. 4 (2016). https://doi.org/10.1371/journal.pone.0152127.

Linnanmäki, L., Kanto, K., Karjalainen, T., Leppänen, O. V., & Lehtinen, J. "Platelet-rich Plasma or Autologous Blood Do Not Reduce Pain or Improve Function in Patients with Lateral Epicondylitis: A Randomized Controlled Trial." *Clinical Orthopaedics and Related Research*, 478(8) (2020), 1892–1900. https://doi.org/10.1097/CORR.0000000000001185

Lorenzo, Serra-Prat, and Yébenes. "The Role of Water Homeostasis in Muscle Function and Frailty: A Review." *Nutrients* 11, no. 8 (2019): 1857. https://doi.org/10.3390/nu11081857.

Mammucari, M., et al. "Mesotherapy: From Historical Notes to Scientific Evidence and Future Prospects." *The Scientific World Journal* 2020 (2020): 1–9. https://doi.org/10.1155/2020/3542848.

Manchester, K. "Louis Pasteur, Fermentation, and a Rival: History of Science." *South African Journal of Science* 103, no. 9 (September 1, 2007): 377–80. https://doi.org/https://hdl.handle.net/10520/EJC96719.

Manchester, Keith L. "Antoine Béchamp: Père de La Biologie. Oui Ou Non?" *Endeavour* 25, no. 2 (2001): 68–73. https://doi.org/10.1016/s0160-9327(00)01361-2.

Marinelli, R., B. Furst, H. van der Zee, A. McGinn, and W. Marinelli. "The Heart Is Not a Pump: A Refutation of the Pressure Propulsion Premise of Heart Function." *Front Perspect* 5, 1995, 1–10.

Marques, M., et al. "Role of Intracellular Water in the Normal-to-Cancer Transition in Human Cells—Insights from Quasi-Elastic Neutron Scattering." *Structural Dynamics* 7, no. 5 (2020). https://doi.org/10.1063/4.0000021.

Mitchell, Jamie R. "Is the Heart a Pressure or Flow Generator? Possible Implications and Suggestions for Cardiovascular Pedagogy." *Advances in Physiology Education* 39, no. 3 (2015): 242–47. https://doi.org/10.1152/advan.00057.2015.

Stopping Pain

Morishita, Kazuhiro, Kengo Watanabe, and Hidenori Ichijo. "Cell Volume Regulation in Cancer Cell Migration Driven by Osmotic Water Flow." *Cancer Science* 110, no. 8 (2019): 2337–47. https://doi.org/10.1111/cas.14079.

Ocasio, Ethan, and Tim Q. Duong. "Deep Learning Prediction of Mild Cognitive Impairment Conversion to Alzheimer's Disease at 3 Years after Diagnosis Using Longitudinal and Whole-Brain 3D MRI." *J Computer Science* 7 (2021). https://doi.org/10.7717/peerj-cs.560.

Pollack, Gerald H. *The Fourth Phase of Water: Beyond Solid, Liquid, and Vapor.* Ebner & Sons, 2013

Pollack, Gerald H., Xavier Figueroa, and Qing Zhao. "The Minimal Cell and Life's Origin: Role of Water and Aqueous Interfaces." *The Minimal Cell*, 2010, 105–21. https://doi.org/10.1007/978-90-481-9944-0_7.

Previtali, D., et al. "The Long-Lasting Effects of 'Placebo Injections' in Knee Osteoarthritis: A Meta-Analysis." *CARTILAGE* 13, no. 1 suppl (2020). https://doi.org/10.1177/1947603520906597.

Qiu, Anqi, Liyuan Xu, and Chaoqiang Liu. "Predicting Diagnosis 4 Years Prior to Alzheimer's Disease Incident." *NeuroImage: Clinical* 34 (2022): 102993. https://doi.org/10.1016/j.nicl.2022.102993.

Quinton, R. *L'Eau de Mer, Milieu Organique.* Masson et Cie, 1912.

Reffitt, D. M., N. Ogston, R. Jugdaohsingh, H. F. J. Cheung, B. A. J. Evans, R. P. H. Thompson, J. J. Powell, and G. N. Hampson. "Orthosilicic Acid Stimulates Collagen Type 1 Synthesis and Osteoblastic Differentiation in Human Osteoblast-like Cells in Vitro." *Bone* 32, no. 2 (2003): 127–35. https://doi.org/10.1016/s8756-3282(02)00950-x.

Rosseland, Leiv A., Knut G. Helgesen, Harald Breivik, and Audun Stubhaug. "Moderate-to-Severe Pain after Knee Arthroscopy Is Relieved by Intraarticular Saline: A Randomized Controlled Trial." *Anesthesia & Analgesia*, 2004, 1546–51. https://doi.org/10.1213/01.ane.0000112433.71197.fa.

Saltzman, B., et al. "The Therapeutic Effect of Intra-Articular Normal Saline Injections for Knee Osteoarthritis: A Meta-Analysis of Evidence Level 1 Studies." *The American Journal of Sports Medicine* 45, no. 11 (2016): 2647–53. https://doi.org/10.1177/0363546516680607.

References

Sarafian, A. R., S. G. Nielsen, H. R. Marschall, F. M. McCubbin, and B. D. Monteleone. "Early Accretion of Water in the Inner Solar System from a Carbonaceous Chondrite-like Source." *Science* 346, no. 6209 (2014): 623–26. https://doi.org/10.1126/science.1256717.

Schultz, Myron. "Rudolf Virchow." *Emerging Infectious Diseases* 14, no. 9 (2008): 1480–81. https://doi.org/10.3201/eid1409.086672.

Simental-Mendía M., Vilchez-Cavazos, F., Álvarez-Villalobos, N., Blázquez-Saldaña, J., Peña-Martínez, V., Villarreal-Villarreal, G., Acosta-Olivo, C. "Clinical efficacy of platelet-rich plasma in the treatment of lateral epicondylitis: a systematic review and meta-analysis of randomized placebo-controlled clinical trials." *Clin Rheumatol*. August 2020; 39 (8):2255-2265. doi: 10.1007/s10067-020-05000-y. Epub 2020 Feb 26. PMID: 32103373.

Sophia Fox, Alice J., Asheesh Bedi, and Scott A. Rodeo. "The Basic Science of Articular Cartilage: Structure, Composition, and Function." *Sports Health* 1, no. 6 (2009): 461–68. https://doi.org/10.1177/1941738109350438.

Szent-Györgyi, Albert. *The Living State: With Observations on Cancer.* Academic Press, 1972.

Trouard, Theodore P., Kevin D. Harkins, Joseph L. Divijak, Robert J. Gillies, and Jean-Philippe Galons. "Ischemia-Induced Changes of Intracellular Water Diffusion in Rat Glioma Cell Cultures." *Magnetic Resonance in Medicine* 60, no. 2 (2008): 258–64. https://doi.org/10.1002/mrm.21616.

Van Putten, M., et al. "Dysregulation of Astrocyte Ion Homeostasis and Its Relevance for Stroke-Induced Brain Damage." *International Journal of Molecular Sciences* 22, no. 11 (2021): 5679. https://doi.org/10.3390/ijms22115679. 34073593; PMCID: PMC8198632.

Vora, Ariana, Joanne Borg-Stein, and Rosalyn T. Nguyen. "Regenerative Injection Therapy for Osteoarthritis: Fundamental Concepts and Evidence-Based Review." *PM&R* 4 (2012). https://doi.org/10.1016/j.pmrj.2012.02.005.

Whitcomb, Isobel. "This Pseudoscience Movement Wants to Wipe Germs from Existence." *Popular Science*, January 3, 2022. https://www.popsci.com/health/germ-theory-terrain-theory/.

Stopping Pain

Yeh, Peter Chia, Shiv Patel, and Rosalyn Nguyen. "Ultrasound-Guided Lavage and Aspiration for Calcific Rotator Cuff Tendinosis." *American Journal of Physical Medicine & Rehabilitation* 99, no. 12 (2020). https://doi.org/10.1097/phm.0000000000001415.

Yelland, Michael J., Paul P. Glasziou, Nikolai Bogduk, Philip J. Schluter, and Mary McKernon. "Prolotherapy Injections, Saline Injections, and Exercises for Chronic Low-Back Pain: A Randomized Trial." *Spine* 29, no. 1 (2004): 9–16. https://doi.org/10.1097/01.brs.0000105529.07222.5b.

Zhang, Na, Jianfen Zhang, Songming Du, and Guansheng Ma. "Dehydration and Rehydration Affect Brain Regional Density and Homogeneity among Young Male Adults, Determined via Magnetic Resonance Imaging: A Pilot Self-Control Trial." *Frontiers in Nutrition* 9 (2022). https://doi.org/10.3389/fnut.2022.906088.

Zhang, W., J. Robertson, A. C. Jones, P. A. Dieppe, and M. Doherty. "The Placebo Effect and Its Determinants in Osteoarthritis: Meta-Analysis of Randomised Controlled Trials." *Annals of the Rheumatic Diseases* 67, no. 12 (2008): 1716–23. https://doi.org/10.1136/ard.2008.092015.

Chapter 6

Boraldi, Federica, Francesco Demetrio Lofaro, and Daniela Quaglino. "Apoptosis in the Extraosseous Calcification Process." *Cells* 10, no. 1 (2021): 131. https://doi.org/10.3390/cells10010131.

Brady, M., and T. George. "Ethylenediaminetetraacetic Acid (EDTA)." In: StatPearls. StatPearls Publishing, June 7, 2022. https://www.ncbi.nlm.nih.gov/books/NBK565883/.

Cacchio, Angelo, Elisabetta De Blasis, Piergiorgio Desiati, Giorgio Spacca, Valter Santilli, and Fosco De Paulis. "Effectiveness of Treatment of Calcific Tendinitis of the Shoulder by Disodium EDTA." *Arthritis Care & Research* 61, no. 1 (2008): 84–91. https://doi.org/10.1002/art.24370.

Constantino, Cosimo, Emilio Marangio, and Gabriella Coruzzi. "Mesotherapy versus Systemic Therapy in the Treatment of Acute Low Back Pain: A Randomized Trial." *Evidence-Based Complementary and Alternative Medicine* 2011 (2011): 1–6. https://doi.org/10.1155/2011/317183.

References

Dalloz-Bourguignon, A. "La Mésothérapie [Mesotherapy]." *Chir Dent Fr*. French 50, no. 76 (September 4, 1980): 43–45. PMID: 6937322.

Dalloz-Bourguignon, André. *Dix Gestes de mésothérapie [Ten Gestures of Mesotherapy]*. Maloine, 1980.

Giordano, C., N. L. Onyinyechi, and C. Sara. "Hypodermoclysis: The Modern Use in Care of an Ancient Therapeutic Technic." *J Hosp Palliat Med Care* 1: 003. (December 18, 2018).

Guez, B. "Mesotherapie de Surface Dans Le Traitment Des Lombalgies: Revue de Cas Cliniques a Propos de 25 Cas (Technique Hydrotmie Percutanee)." 15th Congres International de Mesotherapie. March 29, 2019. https://percutaneoushydrotomy.net/scientific-studies/

Guez, B. "Percutaneous Hydrotomy and Hydro-Mesoperfusion: Chronic Pain, Intractable Osteoarthritis, Aesthetic Medicine." Annual meeting of the Swiss Society of Mesotherapy, October 3, 1998. https://percutaneoushydrotomy.net/scientific-studies/.

Guez, Bernard. *Vaincres Les Maladies Chronique par L'hydrotomie Percutanee*. Dauphin Editions, 2021.

Kim, K. M. "Apoptosis and Calcification." *Scanning Microsc* 9, no. 4 (1995): 1137–75. https://doi.org/PMID: 8819895.

Klein, J. A., and L. J. Langman "Prevention of Surgical Site Infections and Biofilms: Pharmacokinetics of Subcutaneous Cefazolin and Metronidazole in a Tumescent Lidocaine Solution." *Plast Reconstr Surg Glob Open*. May 30, 2017; 5 (5):e1351. doi: 10.1097/GOX.0000000000001351. PMID: 28607871; PMCID: PMC5459654.

Luther, Chelsea A., James L. Griffith, Elena Kurland, Reem Al Shabeeb, Misty Eleryan, Kelley Redbord, and David M. Ozog. "The Infection Rate of Intralesional Triamcinolone and the Safety of Compounding in Dermatology for Intradermal and Subcutaneous Injection: A Retrospective Medical Record Review." *Journal of the American Academy of Dermatology* 83, no. 4 (2020): 1044–48. https://doi.org/10.1016/j.jaad.2020.05.069.

Menkes, C-J., and N. E. Lane. "Are Osteophytes Good or Bad?" *Osteoarthritis and Cartilage* 12 (2004): 53–54. https://doi.org/10.1016/j.joca.2003.09.003.

Nguyen, C. "Treatment of Gonarthrosis: Conventional Mesotherapy versus Percutaneous Hydrotomy, 20 Cases." Dissertation for the interuniversity diploma in mesotherapy (Paris 6 University—La Pitié Salpêtrière), June 2009. https://doi.org/https://percutaneoushydrotomy.net/scientific-studies/.

Pistor, Michel. *Un défi thérapeutique: La Mésothérapie*. Maloine, 1986.

Pitzurra, M., and P. Marconi. "Immunogenesis and Mesotherapy: The Immunoresponse to Antigens Inoculated Intradermally." *Giornale di Mesoterapia* 1 (1981): 9–14.

Sarkar, Rashmi, VijayKumar Garg, and Venkataram Mysore. "Position Paper on Mesotherapy." *Indian Journal of Dermatology, Venereology, and Leprology* 77, no. 2 (2011): 232. https://doi.org/10.4103/0378-6323.77479.

Sears, Margaret E. "Chelation: Harnessing and Enhancing Heavy Metal Detoxification—a Review." *The Scientific World Journal* 2013 (2013): 1–13. https://doi.org/10.1155/2013/219840.

Sivagnanam, G. "Mesotherapy—the French Connection." *Journal of Pharmacology and Pharmacotherapeutics* 1, no. 1 (2010): 4–8. https://doi.org/10.4103/0976-500x.64529.

Vidal, A. L. "Study of 6 Cases of Lumbar Mesoperfusion with Physiological Saline in Large Dilutions for Chronic Low Back Pain, Lumbosciatica." Dissertation for the interuniversity diploma in mesotherapy, University of Bordeaux, June 21, 2019. https://percutaneoushydrotomy.net/scientific-studies/.

Chapter 7

Akbas, Ilker, Meryem Betos Kocak, Abdullah Osman Kocak, Sultan Tuna Gur, Sinem Dogruyol, Mehmet Demir, and Zeynep Cakir. "Intradermal Mesotherapy versus Intravenous Dexketoprofen for the Treatment of Migraine Headache without Aura: A Randomized Controlled Trial." *Annals of Saudi Medicine* 41, no. 3 (2021): 127–34. https://doi.org/10.5144/0256-4947.2021.127.

American Academy of Orthopaedic Surgeons. "One in two Americans have a musculoskeletal condition." *ScienceDaily*, March 1, 2016. www.sciencedaily.com/releases/2016/03/160301114116.htm

References

André Pedro Oliveira Cruz, Ana Filipa Rodrigues das Neves, Isabel Ramires, and Manuel Mendonça. "Effectiveness of Mesotherapy on Temporomandibular Joint Disorders." *Journal of Physical Science and Application* 5, no. 4 (2015). https://doi.org/10.17265/2159-5348/2015.04.001.

Barbara, Giovanni, Cesare Cremon, Giovanni Carini, Lara Bellacosa, Lisa Zecchi, Roberto De Giorgio, Roberto Corinaldesi, and Vincenzo Stanghellini. "The Immune System in Irritable Bowel Syndrome." *Journal of Neurogastroenterology and Motility* 17, no. 4 (2011): 349–59. https://doi.org/10.5056/jnm.2011.17.4.349.

Bedoui, Yosra, Xavier Guillot, Jimmy Sélambarom, Pascale Guiraud, Claude Giry, Marie Christine Jaffar-Bandjee, Stéphane Ralandison, and Philippe Gasque. "Methotrexate an Old Drug with New Tricks." *International Journal of Molecular Sciences* 20, no. 20 (2019): 5023. https://doi.org/10.3390/ijms20205023.

Beutner, C., Wrobel, C., Dombrowski, T., Beutner, D., Forkel, S., Buhl, T. "Inconsistent Skin Prick Tests for Allergy to Birch Homologous Trees May Result from Cross-Reacting Allergens or Technical Errors." *Int Arch Allergy Immunol*. 2023 Jun 2:1-8. doi: 10.1159/000530201.

Birkhoff, M., M. Leitz, and D. Marx. "Advantages of Intranasal Vaccination and Considerations on Device Selection." *Indian Journal of Pharmaceutical Sciences* 71, no. 6 (2009): 729–31.

Bunker, Tim D. "Frozen Shoulder." Oxford Medicine Online, 2011. https://doi.org/10.1093/med/9780199550647.003.004005.

Burch, Rebecca C., Stephen Loder, Elizabeth Loder, and Todd A. Smitherman. "The Prevalence and Burden of Migraine and Severe Headache in the United States: Updated Statistics from Government Health Surveillance Studies." *Headache* 55, no. 1 (2015): 21–34. https://doi.org/10.1111/head.12482.

Cacchio, A., et al. "Effectiveness of Treatment of Calcific Tendinitis of the Shoulder by Disodium EDTA." *Arthritis Care & Research* 61, no. 1 (2008): 84–91. https://doi.org/10.1002/art.24370.

Campbell, James N., and Richard A. Meyer. "Mechanisms of Neuropathic Pain." *Neuron* 52, no. 1 (2006): 77–92. https://doi.org/10.1016/j.neuron.2006.09.021.

Stopping Pain

Caputi, Claudio A., and Vincenzo Firetto. "Therapeutic Blockade of Greater Occipital and Supraorbital Nerves in Migraine Patients." *Headache* 37, no. 3 (1997): 174–79. https://doi.org/10.1046/j.1526-4610.1997.3703174.x.

Cho, Bo Young, Judith Murovic, Kyung Woo Park, and Jon Park. "Lumbar Disc Rehydration Postimplantation of a Posterior Dynamic Stabilization System." *Journal of Neurosurgery: Spine* 13, no. 5 (2010): 576–80. https://doi.org/10.3171/2010.5.spine08418.

Combadiere, Behazine, and Christelle Liard. "Transcutaneous and Intradermal Vaccination." *Human Vaccines* 7, no. 8 (2011): 811–27. https://doi.org/10.4161/hv.7.8.16274.

Cross, Marita, Emma Smith, Damian Hoy, Sandra Nolte, Ilana Ackerman, Marlene Fransen, Lisa Bridgett, et al. "The Global Burden of Hip and Knee Osteoarthritis: Estimates from the Global Burden of Disease 2010 Study." *Annals of the Rheumatic Diseases* 73, no. 7 (2014): 1323–30. https://doi.org/10.1136/annrheumdis-2013-204763.

De Carli, Angelo, Ferdinando Pulcinelli, Giacomo Rose, Dario Pitino, and Andrea Ferretti. "Calcific Tendinitis of the Shoulder." *Joints* 02, no. 03 (2014): 130–36. https://doi.org/10.11138/jts/2014.2.3.130.

Edwards, J. "Successful Case of Percutaneous Hydrotomy for the Shoulder in a UFC Athlete." Annual meeting of the International Society of Percutaneous Hydrotomy, 2021.

Faas, M. M., and P. de Vos. "Mitochondrial Function in Immune Cells in Health and Disease." *Biochimica et Biophysica Acta (BBA)—Molecular Basis of Disease* 1866, no. 10 (2020): 165845. https://doi.org/10.1016/j.bbadis.2020.165845.

Freburger, Janet K., George M. Holmes, Robert P. Agans, Anne M. Jackman, Jane D. Darter, Andrea S. Wallace, Liana D. Castel, William D. Kalsbeek, and Timothy S. Carey. "The Rising Prevalence of Chronic Low Back Pain." *Archives of Internal Medicine* 169, no. 3 (2009): 251. https://doi.org/10.1001/archinternmed.2008.543.

Granville-Smith, Isabelle, Nathan P. Danckert, Maxim B. Freidin, Philippa Wells, Julian R. Marchesi, and Frances M. Williams. "Evidence for Infection in Intervertebral Disc Degeneration: A Systematic Review."

References

European Spine Journal 31, no. 2 (2021): 414–30. https://doi.org/10.1007/s00586-021-07062-1.

Guez, Bernard. *Vaincres Les Maladies Chronique par l'Hydrotomie Percutanee.* Dauphin Editions, 2021.

Hassan, Amal Ali, Mona Hamdy Nasr, Ahmed Lotfi Mohamed, Ahmed Mohmed Kamal, and Alyaa Diaa Elmoghazy. "Psychological Affection in Rheumatoid Arthritis Patients in Relation to Disease Activity." *Medicine* 98, no. 19 (2019). https://doi.org/10.1097/md.0000000000015373.

Kim, Malin. "Saline Injections for Prophylactic Treatment of Chronic Migraine—Ongoing Study." Case Medical Research—Göteborg University, 2019. https://doi.org/10.31525/ct1-nct03919045.

Kuo, D. T. and P. Tadi *Cervical Spondylosis.* May 1, 2023. PMID: 31855384. StatPearls Publishing.

Lemaire, Y. "'Advantage of Large Dilutions in Mesotherapy in the Clinical Management of Chronic Cervicogenic Headaches.'" Dissertation for the interuniversity diploma in Mesotherapy—Bordeaux, June 2016. https://doi.org/https://percutaneoushydrotomy.net/scientific-studies/.

Levin, Morris. "Nerve Blocks in the Treatment of Headache." *Neurotherapeutics* 7, no. 2 (2010): 197–203. https://doi.org/10.1016/j.nurt.2010.03.001.

Li, Dion Tik, and Yiu Yan Leung. "Temporomandibular Disorders: Current Concepts and Controversies in Diagnosis and Management." *Diagnostics* 11, no. 3 (2021): 459. https://doi.org/10.3390/diagnostics11030459.

Linetsky, Felix S., Rafael Miguel, and Francisco Torres. "Treatment of Cervicothoracic Pain and Cervicogenic Headaches with Regenerative Injection Therapy." *Current Pain and Headache Reports* 8, no. 1 (2004): 41–48. https://doi.org/10.1007/s11916-004-0039-3.

Longstreth, George F., W. Grant Thompson, William D. Chey, Lesley A. Houghton, Fermin Mearin, and Robin C. Spiller. "Functional Bowel Disorders." *Gastroenterology* 130, no. 5 (2006): 1480–91. https://doi.org/10.1053/j.gastro.2005.11.061.

Luime, J. J., B. W. Koes, I. J. M. Hendriksen, A. Burdorf, A. P. Verhagen, H. S. Miedema, and J. A. N. Verhaar. "Prevalence and Incidence of Shoulder Pain in the General Population; a Systematic Review." *Scandinavian*

Journal of Rheumatology 33, no. 2 (2004): 73–81. https://doi.org/10.1080/03009740310004667.

Maeda, Kazuhiko, Matias J. Caldez, and Shizuo Akira. "Innate Immunity in Allergy." *Allergy* 74, no. 9 (2019): 1660–74. https://doi.org/10.1111/all.13788.

Mammucari M., et al. "Mesotherapy: From Historical Notes to Scientific Evidence and Future Prospects." *Scientific World Journal*. 2020 May 1;2020:3542848. doi: 10.1155/2020/3542848. PMID: 32577099; PMCID: PMC7305548.

Manske, Robert C., and Daniel Prohaska. "Diagnosis and Management of Adhesive Capsulitis." *Current Reviews in Musculoskeletal Medicine* 1, no. 3–4 (2008): 180–89. https://doi.org/10.1007/s12178-008-9031-6.

Marynowski, Mateusz. "Role of Environmental Pollution in Irritable Bowel Syndrome." *World Journal of Gastroenterology* 21, no. 40 (2015): 11371. https://doi.org/10.3748/wjg.v21.i40.11371.

Meloche JP, Bergeron Y, Bellavance A, Morand M, Huot J, Belzile G. "Painful intervertebral dysfunction: Robert Maigne's original contribution to headache of cervical origin." The Quebec Headache Study Group. *Headache*. June 1993; 33 (6):328-34. doi: 10.1111/j.1526-4610.1993.hed3306328.x. PMID: 8349476.

Mobasheri, Ali, and Mark Batt. "An Update on the Pathophysiology of Osteoarthritis." *Annals of Physical and Rehabilitation Medicine* 59, no. 5–6 (2016): 333–39. https://doi.org/10.1016/j.rehab.2016.07.004.

Netea, Mihai G., Jorge Domínguez-Andrés, Luis B. Barreiro, Triantafyllos Chavakis, Maziar Divangahi, Elaine Fuchs, Leo A. Joosten, et al. "Defining Trained Immunity and Its Role in Health and Disease." *Nature Reviews Immunology* 20, no. 6 (2020): 375–88. https://doi.org/10.1038/s41577-020-0285-6.

Nicolas, Jean-François, and Bruno Guy. "Intradermal, Epidermal and Transcutaneous Vaccination: From Immunology to Clinical Practice." *Expert Review of Vaccines* 7, no. 8 (2008): 1201–14. https://doi.org/10.1586/14760584.7.8.1201.

Noël, E., T. Thomas, T. Schaeverbeke, P. Thomas, M. Bonjean, and M. Revel. "Frozen Shoulder." *Joint Bone Spine* 67, no. 5 (2000): 393–400.

References

Ramachandran, R., & Yaksh, T. L. "Therapeutic use of botulinum toxin in migraine: mechanisms of action." *British Journal of Pharmacology*, 171(18) (2014), 4177–4192. https://doi.org/10.1111/bph.12763

Ramirez, J. "Adhesive Capsulitis: Diagnosis and Management." *Am Fam Physician* 99, no. 5 (March 1, 2019): 297–300. https://doi.org/PMID: 30811157.

Roush, J. K., R. M. McLaughlin, and M. Radlinsky. "Understanding the Pathophysiology of Osteoarthritis." *Veterinary Medicine* 97, no. 2 (2002): 108–17.

Soncini, G, and C. Constantino. "Il Trattamento Delle Tendinopatie Calcifiche Di Spalla Con E.D.T.A. Sale Bisodico per via Mesoterapica [The Treatment of Pathologic Calcification of Shoulder Tendons with E.D.T.A. Bisodium Salt by Mesotherapy]." *Acta Biomed Ateneo Parmense.* Italian. 69, no. 5–6 (1998): 133–38. https://doi.org/PMID: 10702841.

Sparks, Jeffrey A. "Rheumatoid Arthritis." *Annals of Internal Medicine* 170, no. 1 (2019). https://doi.org/10.7326/aitc201901010.

Taylor, A., and G. McLeod. "Basic Pharmacology of Local Anaesthetics." *BJA Education* 20, no. 2 (2020): 34–41. https://doi.org/10.1016/j.bjae.2019.10.002.

Tepper, Stewart J. "A Pivotal Moment in 50 Years of Headache History: The First American Migraine Study." *Headache* 48, no. 5 (2008): 730–31. https://doi.org/10.1111/j.1526-4610.2008.01117_1.x.

Volinn, E., and J. D. Loeser. "What Are the Origins of Chronic Back Pain of 'Obscure Origins'? Turning toward Family and Workplace Social Contexts." *The Yale Journal of Biology and Medicine* 95, no. 1 (March 31, 2022): 153–63. https://doi.org/PMID: 35370485.

Vos, Theo, Ryan M. Barber, Brad Bell, Amelia Bertozzi-Villa, Stan Biryukov, Ian Bolliger, Fiona Charlson, et al. "Global, Regional, and National Incidence, Prevalence, and Years Lived with Disability for 301 Acute and Chronic Diseases and Injuries in 188 Countries, 1990–2013: A Systematic Analysis for the Global Burden of Disease Study 2013." *The Lancet* 386, no. 9995 (2015): 743–800. https://doi.org/10.1016/s0140-6736(15)60692-4.

Yamamoto, Erin A., and Trine N. Jørgensen. "Relationships between Vitamin D, Gut Microbiome, and Systemic Autoimmunity." *Frontiers in Immunology* 10 (2020). https://doi.org/10.3389/fimmu.2019.03141.

Yasuda, Takuwa, Takehiro Ura, Masaru Taniguchi, and Hisahiro Yoshida. "Intradermal Delivery of Antigens Enhances Specific IGG and Diminishes IGE Production: Potential Use for Vaccination and Allergy Immunotherapy." *PLOS ONE* 11, no. 12 (2016). https://doi.org/10.1371/journal.pone.0167952.

Yilmaz, Attila, Salim Senturk, Mehdi Sasani, Tunc Oktenoglu, Onur Yaman, Hakan Yildirim, Tuncer Suzer, and Ali Fahir Ozer. "Disc Rehydration after Dynamic Stabilization: A Report of 59 Cases." *Asian Spine Journal* 11, no. 3 (2017): 348–55. https://doi.org/10.4184/asj.2017.11.3.348.

Chapter 8

Edwards, J. "Successful Case of Percutaneous Hydrotomy for the Shoulder in a UFC Athlete." Annual meeting of the International Society of Percutaneous Hydrotomy, 2021.

Guez, B. "Case Presentations and New Treatments in Percutaneous Hydrotomy." Annual meeting of the International Society of Percutaneous Hydrotomy, 2021.

Guez, Bernard. *Vaincres Les Maladies Chronique par L'hydrotomie Percutanee*. Dauphin Editions, 2021.

Hashemi, S, A Hajiaghajani, and A Abdolali. "Noninvasive Blockade of Action Potential by Electromagnetic Induction." https://arxiv.org/ftp/arxiv/papers/1809/1809.06199.pdf. Accessed August 17, 2023.

Kaplan, A., et al. "Mesoscintigraphy: Contribution of the Meso Technique to Diagnostic Scintigraphy. Pharmacokinetic Implications." 5th International Congress of Mesotherapy, Paris, October 7, 1988.

Lastes, V. "Percutaneous Hydrotomy in Canine & Feline Veterinary Medicine." Annual meeting of the International Society of Percutaneous Hydrotomy, 2019.

Saussey, A. "News in Percutaneous Hydrotomy in Equine Veterinary Medicine." Annual meeting of the International Society of Percutaneous Hydrotomy, 2021.

References

Sivagnanam, G. "Mesotherapy—the French Connection." *Journal of Pharmacology and Pharmacotherapeutics* 1, no. 1 (2010): 4–8. https://doi.org/10.4103/0976-500x.64529.

World Anti-Doping Agency (WADA). The 2022 Prohibited List International Standard. (www.wada-ama.org).

Ye, Hui, Jenna Hendee, Joyce Ruan, Alena Zhirova, Jayden Ye, and Maria Dima. "Neuron Matters: Neuromodulation with Electromagnetic Stimulation Must Consider Neurons as Dynamic Identities." *Journal of NeuroEngineering and Rehabilitation* 19, no. 1 (2022). https://doi.org/10.1186/s12984-022-01094-4.

Chapter 10

Shiple, Brian, and Marlisle Wind. *Regenerative Healing for Life*. Self-published, 2013.

Index

Abramson, John, 33
adhesive capsulitis, 60, 121
aesthetic medicine, 56, 59
agriculture, 27, 29
allergies, 77, 134–135, 176–178
anesthesia, 9, 42, 43, 48, 50, 56, 57, 92, 112, 113, 151
autoimmune, 30, 76, 77, 100, 133, 137, 179

bacteria, 27, 30, 76, 80, 101, 102, 136
Bernard, Claude, 46, 99, 101, 103, 115
Bernard Guez, 7, 9, 13, 49, 169, 178, 184
Bezos, Jeff 28
Biden, Joe 29
Billat, Veronique, 18
biological terrain, 16, 53, 67, 76, 99–103, 115, 116

Calavitta, Sam, 11
California, 11, 29
cancer, 29, 30, 70, 76, 77, 83, 89, 151
chronic disease, 4, 6, 17, 22–31, 61, 70, 72, 87, 88, 96, 98, 100, 102, 116
circadian pollutants, 28
Claude Bernard, 13, 46, 99, 101, 103, 115
copper, 54, 55, 69
corticosteroids, 36, 76, 95, 104, 105, 108, 127, 129–132, 135, 145, 165, 178

COVID-19, 15, 99, 100, 149

depression, 20, 23, 25, 39, 84, 100, 117, 120, 131
Dillashaw, T.J., 18, 123, 124, 144
disability, 8, 23, 116, 117, 125
disease, 4, 6, 17, 19, 22–31, 41, 42, 61, 65, 70, 72, 77, 87, 88, 97, 100, 102, 103, 110, 115, 116, 126, 131, 142, 178, 179
double-blind study, 38

EBM, 37–39
EDTA, 14, 70, 105–107, 112, 121–123, 128, 130, 145, 147
evidence-based-medicine, 37–39

farming, 30
FDA, 32–34, 51, 105, 145, 152
Fournier, Pierre François 56

gabapentin, 36
Gates, Bill 29
Guez, Bernard, 7, 9, 13, 49, 169, 178, 184

herniated disc, 12, 71, 73, 112, 116, 126, 129, 144, 165–168
hydrotomy cushion, 59, 95, 96, 106, 124, 128
hypodermoclysis, 9, 43, 50, 57–58, 106, 113, 153, 181

Index

Illouz, Yves-Gerard, 56
immune system, 29, 30, 65, 75–78, 80, 81, 99–101, 109, 131, 134–138

ketamine, 58
Klein, Jeffrey, 9, 56, 57, 105
kwashiorkor, 12, 42, 44

Lavoisier, Antoine, 46
longevity, 13, 28

Merck, 32–34
mesochelation, 105–108, 111, 119, 121, 123, 126, 128–130, 156–160, 165, 168–171, 173–174
mesoperfusion, 107–109, 128, 129, 161, 162, 165, 167, 168
mesotherapy, 8–10, 42, 43, 48, 49–53, 57, 61, 105, 112, 113, 118, 121–123, 146, 147
mesovaccination, 77–81, 109–110, 132, 136, 138, 175–179
methotrexate, 55, 131, 179
migraine headaches, 22, 24, 84
migraines, 9, 72, 117–120, 156–158
morphine, 47, 58, 156, 157
Musk, Elon, 28, 29

NEJM, 33–34
NSAID, 6, 32, 33, 36, 52, 121, 122, 127, 131, 152

Obama, Barack, 29
obesity, 5, 30, 100, 102, 127, 190
oligotherapy, 7, 9, 43, 49, 53–55, 70, 181
osteoporosis, 36, 72

Pasteur, Louis, 46, 80, 101–103
phosphatidylcholine, 56
Picard, Henry, 54, 69
Pistor, Michel, 10, 16, 48, 50–53, 113, 143, 151
placebo, 97–98
procaine, 48, 50, 121–124, 133, 134, 174

Quinton, René, 12, 16, 43–46, 57, 87, 96

reductionism, 31
Reuben, Scott, 33–34
rheumatoid arthritis, 26, 55, 75, 84, 116, 131–133

selenium, 55, 69
silicium, 95, 110
sport injuries, 10, 144, 172
Szent-Györgyi, Albert, 19, 82, 86, 94, 125

tinnitus, 51, 72, 82, 125, 130
Trump, Donald, 20, 29
tumescent anesthesia, 9, 43, 50, 56, 57, 112, 113, 181
Tylenol, 35

UFC, 17, 18, 123, 144, 188
University of Claude Bernard, 13

Veronique Billat, 18
Vioxx, 32–34, 36
viruses, 30, 76, 80, 81, 101, 102, 136

zinc, 55, 69

About the Author

Dr. Johnathan Edwards

Dr. Johnathan Edwards is a board-certified anesthesiologist who treats chronic pain patients. He was the first American physician to complete his training in percutaneous hydrotomy with Dr. Guez and bring the technique to the United States, and has performed percutaneous hydrotomy on hundreds of patients. He wrote this book to increase interest in percutaneous hydrotomy in the United States and other English-speaking countries worldwide. In conjunction with Dr. Guez and the ISPH, Dr. Edwards has trained many practitioners in the art and science of percutaneous hydrotomy.

Dr. Edwards is the author of several books and medical papers, including *The Revolutionary Ketamine*; *Chasing Dakar*; *Suicide, COVID-19, and Ketamine*; and *The Science of the Marathon*. He practices medicine in Las Vegas, Nevada, and Port Orange, Florida. A native of California, he studied at Victor Valley Community College, the University of California at Davis, and Eastern Virginia Medical School. He later completed training in Lyon, France.

About the Author

Dr. Edwards lives with his wife and their daughter in Port Orange, Florida, and also part-time in the Provence region of France.

For more information, please visit:
www.percutaneoushydrotomy.net
www.johnathanedwardsmd.com